It's Not Just A Swelling!

LYMPHEDEMA

Causes, Prevention, Treatment, Self-Management

Joachim E. Zuther

Lymphedema Specialist, Founder Academy of Lymphatic Studies, Author of the textbook *Lymphedema Management, A Comprehensive Guide For Practitioners* (Thieme Medical Publishers)

Publisher: Prolymph Consultants

ISBN 979-8-9860403-0-1

Also available as e-Book:

eISBN 979-8-9860403-1-8

Introduction

I have been involved in lymphedema care for the past thirty five years, having received my training in Germany, where Complete Decongestive Therapy (CDT) for the treatment and management of lymphedema has been well established since the 1970s.

After relocating to the US in the early 1990s I learned that in this country adequate lymphedema care was not a well-known part of the medical field; there were a handful of treatment centers scattered throughout the country, and institutions for the training and education of health care practitioners in lymphedema management were basically non-existent. Back in those days I was also talking to a large number of physicians about lymphedema and was surprised to learn that the vast majority of these doctors, even specialists such as vascular surgeons and oncologists, did not know what lymphedema was, or how it should be treated. I was even told that lymphedema was a "non-issue" in the US and a "European problem". Patients with lymphedematous extremities were told that there is nothing that could be done and that they would have to live with their swollen arms or legs.

Thankfully this situation has improved over the past decades; many lymphedema treatment centers are now established throughout the country, and there are a number of excellent schools providing high quality training in lymphedema management to health care practitioners.

CDT is now recognized in the United States as the gold standard treatment for lymphedema, and health care providers generally do a good job in providing information on this condition and how to best avoid it following surgical procedures.

With the development of the Internet we also saw the evolution of a large number of websites dedicated to lymphedema and its care, providing patients affected by lymphedema with the information they need, which is of great importance especially for those patients who do not receive adequate information from their physicians and caregivers.

Progress has also been made in alternative or additional treatment modalities for lymphedema, such as surgical procedures and new generation intermittent pneumatic compression devices (PCDs).

Various surgical procedures for the treatment of lymphedema have been practiced for over a century and advancements in medical technologies have led to increased discussion of the role surgical treatment, such as lympho-lymphatic or lympho-venous anastomoses and vascularized lymph node transfers.

Recent research indicates that the surgical approach to treat lymphedema has beneficial effects for a select group of patients; however, there is a broad consensus that surgical procedures do not eliminate the need of CDT pre- as well as post-operatively, and should act as an adjunct to conservative treatment protocols. Any surgical approach to treat lymphedema should be reserved for those cases when conservative treatments have clearly been unsuccessful or when the achieved success of conservative measures can no longer be maintained.

An important component to determine whether any surgical procedure for lymphedema is indicated is to weigh the potential benefit of the specific surgical procedure against the risks associated with it. Other considerations should include the individual needs and goals of the patient, and the medical expertise of the surgical team.

Recent studies suggest that there is a potential place for newer generation intermittent pneumatic compression pumps (PCDs) as a beneficial adjunct treatment to control lymphedema, specifically for individuals affected by chronic lymphedema with limited or no access to medical care, or in those cases when physical limitations of the individual may result in challenges controlling the lymphedema independently in the self-administered maintenance phase directly following CDT treatments.

It is important to point out that PCDs should not be used as a stand-alone therapy for lymphedema, and that compression therapy with bandages and/or garments must be continued following the use of PCDs to prevent a rebound of swelling. Optimal treatment and management of lymphedema always necessitates a treatment approach that is tailored to the patient's specific needs. PCD devices can be an additional tool in a multi-modality approach to effectively treat lymphedema; however, no pneumatic compression device is able to replace Complete Decongestive Therapy.

Lymphedema management in the US has certainly evolved; many outstanding researchers, educators and individuals involved in the field are constantly working to further improve lymphedema care. However, continued improvement is needed in areas such as the education of physicians and other health care providers in the effective treatment of lymphedema (the lymphatic system is hardly covered in medical school), health care coverage for compression garments and research on the impact of early and late onset lymphedema on the psycho-social and functional health of affected patients.

It is my hope that this book will provide increased awareness and understanding of this often-neglected condition and serve as a helpful guide in navigating important aspects of lymphedema care and management for individuals affected by lymphedema, their family members and caregivers.

Joachim E. Zuther

Table of Contents

1.0 Lymphatic System

1.1 Function

The lymphatic system is part of the circulatory network and is a vital component of the immune system. It can be thought of as a secondary circulatory system that runs in conjunction and parallel with the cardiovascular system, and consists of a network of lymphatic vessels that carry a clear fluid known as lymph (from Latin: lympha = water).

In addition to vessels, the lymphatic system includes lymphoid organs, which can be divided into primary and secondary categories. The bone marrow and thymus are primary organs responsible for the production and maturation of T and B lymphocytes, which will then colonize the secondary, peripheral organs, such as the lymph nodes, tonsils, spleen, and Peyer's patches (small lymphatic organs) in the small intestine.

Secondary lymphatic organs are laid out as a series of filters, which monitor and filter the components of the lymph fluid and blood. Lymphocytes residing in these organs are positioned to initiate appropriate immune responses.

The lymphatic system has multiple interrelated functions:

- Collection and transport of fluids from all body tissues back to the venous system. By removing fluids that are forced out from the blood vessels, it maintains normal fluid levels within the tissues (fluid homeostasis).
- Absorption and transportation of fatty acids from the digestive system.
- Removal of cellular waste, such as dead cells, bacteria, toxins and other impurities.
- Immune response; lymph nodes and other lymphatic organs filter the lymph to remove microorganisms and other foreign particles.

Without adequate drainage, excess body fluids can accumulate in the tissues, resulting in swelling known as either edema or lymphedema.

1.2 Structural Components of the Lymphatic System

1.2.1 Lymph Nodes

Lymph nodes are soft round, kidney or bean-shaped structures that are an integral part of the immune system filtering lymph, the clear fluid that circulates through the lymphatic system. They drain lymph fluid from nearby organs or areas of the body (tributary or drainage areas) and become swollen in response to infection and malignancies.

The majority of lymph nodes are embedded in fatty tissue and are arranged in either groups (regional lymph nodes) or chains; their normal size in adults is less than half inch (generally 0.2 to 0.3 cm). In case of infections or malignancies, lymph nodes can increase in size.

The number of lymph nodes in an average human varies between 600 and 700; a set number of lymph nodes is present at the time of birth and while their size increases and decreases during the course of life, lymph nodes do not regenerate or disappear.

Clusters of lymph nodes are found in the neck, underarm (axilla), chest, abdomen, and groin; for example, there are about 20-40 lymph nodes in the axilla (Fig. 1.3).

Most nodes are strategically located in places where pathogens enter, such as the head-neck area and the intestines.

Function

Lymph nodes play an essential role in the body's immune defense by filtering harmful material (cancer cells, pathogens) entering the lymph nodes and producing antigen-stimulated lymphocytes, also known as antibodies. Antibodies leave the lymph nodes and travel within the lymph fluid to the blood and are then distributed throughout the body to defend against foreign invaders.

Lymph fluid enters the lymph nodes through incoming (afferent) lymph collectors, which perforate the capsular area, and leaves the nodes at an area known as the hilus via outgoing lymph (efferent) collectors; lymph collectors also connect different lymph nodes with each other.

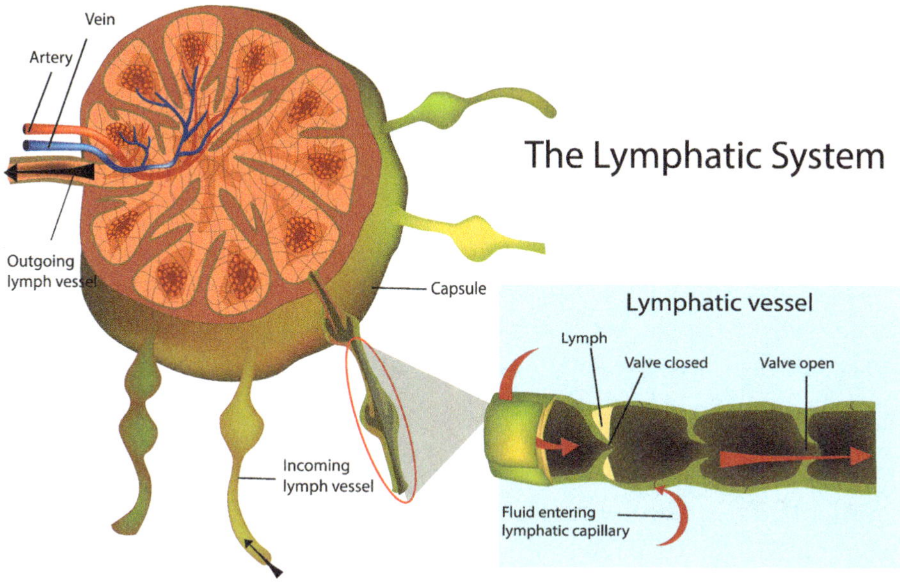

Figure 1.1 Cross section of a lymph node with afferent and efferent lymph vessels

In order to ensure adequate monitoring and filter function, lymph fluid will pass, in most cases, through more than one lymph node before it returns to the blood circulation.

Extensions of the capsular area of lymph nodes consist of connective tissue, which provides support for blood vessels entering into the nodes; this connective tissue compartmentalizes the inside of the lymph node into sinus systems, in which lymph fluid slowly circulates within the lymph node (Fig. 1.1).

In many cases, regional lymph nodes represent the first line of defense in the lymph transport. The drainage or tributary area of a group of regional lymph nodes may include several lymphatic territories. For example, the tributary area for the lymph nodes located in the groin (inguinal lymph nodes) consists of the legs, the buttocks, or gluteal area, the skin of the external genitalia, perineum, and the lower body quadrants (abdominal and lumbar areas below the naval line). The tributary area for the axillary lymph nodes includes the arms and the upper body quadrants (chest and back above the naval line).

Lymph Nodes and Metastases

Cancer can either start in lymph nodes, in which case it would be known as lymphoma, or it can spread there from somewhere else. When cancer cells break away from a primary tumor site, they can travel to other areas of the body through either the bloodstream or the lymph system. If they travel through the lymph system, the cancer cells may end up in lymph nodes. Most of the escaped cancer cells die or are killed by defense cells before they can start growing somewhere else; however, some might settle in a new area, begin to grow, and form new tumors. This spread of cancer to a new part of the body is known as *metastasis*.

When cancer does spread to lymph nodes, it usually spreads to nodes near the tumor itself. These are the nodes that have been doing most of the work to filter out or kill the invading cancer cells.

The most common symptom of cancer in the lymph nodes is that one or more lymph nodes become swollen or feel hard, sometimes these nodes even become visible. The swelling or enlargement is called *lymphadenopathy*. If swollen lymph nodes are located inside the chest or deep in the abdominal area, the lymph nodes cannot be seen or felt. Often there are no symptoms. But sometimes swollen lymph nodes may press on nearby organs or structures, which then can cause symptoms. In these cases, doctors may use scans or other imaging tests to look for enlarged nodes that are located deep in the body.

Secondary cancer in the lymph nodes may be diagnosed at the same time as the primary cancer. It may also be found during routine tests and scans after treatment. When cancer is present in a lymph node, a biopsy (samples of one or more nodes using needles) helps determine what type of cancer it is when the removed tissue or node is examined under a microscope. The cancer cells will look like the cancer cells of the tumor where they originated, so breast cancer cells in the lymphatic system will still look like breast cancer.

When a surgeon operates to remove a primary cancer, they may remove one or more of the nearby (regional) lymph nodes as well. Removal of part of one lymph node is known as a *biopsy;* when several lymph nodes are removed, it's called *lymph node dissection.* When cancer has spread to lymph nodes, there is a higher risk that the cancer might come back after surgery. This information helps the physician decide whether more treatment, such as chemotherapy, immunotherapy, or radiation might be needed following the surgical removal.

When lymph nodes are removed, it can leave the affected area without a way to drain away the lymph fluid. Many of the lymph vessels now run into a dead end where the node used to be, and fluid can back up.

This may result in lymphedema, which can become a life-long problem. As a general rule, the higher the number of removed lymph nodes, the more likely lymphedema is to occur.

1.2.2 Lymphatic Vessels

Lymphatic vessels, which are also known as lymphatics, can be categorized as lymph capillaries, or initial lymph vessels, precollectors, collectors, and lymphatic trunks. Lymph vessels are found throughout the body in all areas where there is blood supply, to include the central nervous system (CNS).

Interestingly, lymph vessels in the CNS remained undiscovered until 2015[1,2]; before this time, it was thought that the CNS was deficient of lymphatic vessels. Subsequent research based on this discovery suggests that a disruption of lymphatic pathways may be involved in neurological disorders associated with immune system dysfunctions, such as Autism, Alzheimer's and Parkinson's disease, Multiple Sclerosis and Meningitis. Research suggests that lymphatic clearance of the brain using Manual Lymph Drainage techniques on the deep cervical lymph nodes may play an important role in improving brain lymphatic drainage, possibly resulting in a decrease of neuro-inflammation that is typical in these neurological disorders[3-6].

Capillaries

Lymphatic capillaries (20-70 μm in diameter) represent the beginning of the lymphatic drainage system, which is why these vessels are also referred to in the literature as *initial lymph vessels*. The main function of capillaries is the absorption of lymph fluid (Lymphatic Loads, Page 12), which is known as *lymph formation*. Lymph capillaries originate in close proximity to blood capillaries as closed or dead-end tubes in the tissue spaces below the skin (sub-endothelial layers) and in the mucous membranes (Fig. 1.2).

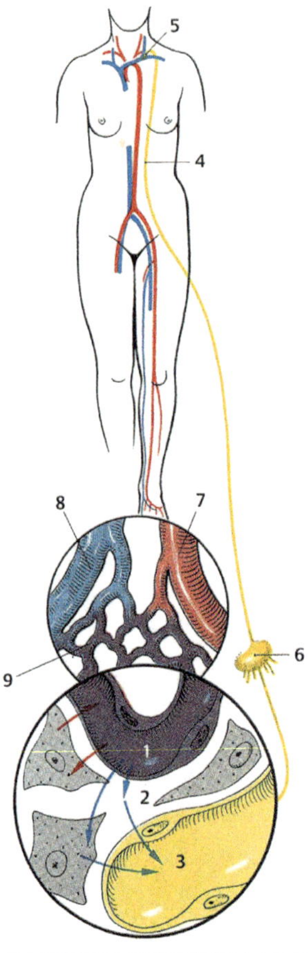

Fig. 1.2 Lymphatic return 1, blood capillary; 2, tissue space; 3, lymph capillary; 4, large lymph vessel; 5, left venous angle; 6, lymph node; 7, artery; 8; vein; 9, blood capillaries. From Kahle, Leonhardt, Platzer Color Atlas/Text Human Anatomy, Vol. 2: Internal Organs. 4th ed. Thieme; 1993) Reprinted with permission

The lymph capillaries of the superficial lymphatic system are connected to each other and form a network covering the entire surface of the body. The meshes of this network are finer in the areas of the fingers, palms, and soles of the feet.

Lymph capillaries resemble blood capillaries but have distinct differences. The lymph capillaries are slightly larger, have a more irregular inner lumen, and are more pervious than blood capillaries, allowing more fluid to pass through their walls. Because of their unique structure, lymph capillaries can absorb large molecules, for example proteins and cell debris.

The flat endothelial cells of lymph capillaries are arranged in a single layer and the links between their cells may have a continuous connection, lay adjacent to each other, or overlap each other like roof tiles. The overlapping structures of the endothelial cells create inlet valves; this structural adaptation ensures the absorption and return of protein, water, and other large molecular substances back into the blood circulatory system.

Fine semi-elastic filaments, also referred to in the literature as anchoring filaments, connect the microfiber network located in the sub-endothelial layer of the lymph capillaries with the surrounding connective tissue; this enables the lymph capillaries to stay open even under high tissue pressure.

When fluid accumulates in the tissues, the fibers of the connective tissue are stretched away from each other, causing a pull on the anchoring filaments that connect the lymph capillaries with the surrounding fiber network. The anchoring filaments then transfer this force to the lymph capillary, which in turn will dilate and cause the endothelial cells of lymph capillaries to open like inlet valves.

The difference in pressure between the inner lumen of the lymph capillary (lower pressure) and the surrounding tissue (higher pressure) creates a suction effect, facilitating the movement of tissue fluid and other components from the tissue spaces into the lymphatic system.

This directional flow of fluid into the lymph capillaries ends when the capillary is filled; in this phase, the pressure inside the lymph capillary is equal or greater than the pressure in the surrounding tissues, which causes the inlet valves of the lymph capillaries to close.

External mobilization of the connective tissue (see also Treatment Chapter; Manual Lymph Drainage) can also manipulate the anchoring filaments, resulting in opening of lymph capillaries, thereby increasing the uptake of tissue fluid into the lymphatic system.

Lymph capillaries do not contain valves, like larger lymph vessels and veins, which enables the lymph fluid to move freely in all directions throughout the initial lymph capillary network. Under normal conditions, lymph fluid moves from the capillaries into the precollectors because the resistance in the somewhat bigger precollectors is lower than in the lymph capillaries.

Precollectors

Lymph capillaries connect to precollectors (70-150 µm in diameter) in the deeper layers of the skin. They constitute the connection and facilitate the transport of lymph fluid between lymphatic capillaries and lymph collectors. The walls of precollectors resemble the lymph capillaries, however, their endothelial cells have predominantly tight connections, and smooth musculature is present in some areas of the walls.

The main function of precollectors is to regulate the flow of lymph fluid unidirectionally from the superficial to the deeper layers of the lymphatic vessel system, which is represented by collectors.

Collectors

Lymph collectors (150-600 µm in diameter) transport lymph fluid to the lymph nodes and the lymphatic trunks. These vessels run horizontally in the fatty layer of the subcutaneous tissue and are larger than lymph capillaries and precollectors.

Lymph collectors have a three-layered wall, similar to veins, which are made of endothelial cells (inner wall), smooth muscle cells (medium layer), and collagen tissue (outer wall). Collectors are categorized into superficial and deep vessels, depending on their location relative to the deep fascia of the body. The collectors below the fascia tend to accompany larger blood vessels, although the superficial collectors in the fatty layer of the skin (above the fascia), which outnumber the deep collectors, have no such preference.

Collectors contain valves, which allow the flow of fluid in one direction only towards lymph nodes and larger lymph collectors, known as trunks (Fig. 1.4). The interval between the valves is irregular and varies between 6 and 20 mm (up to 10 cm in larger trunks).

The segment of a collector located between two pairs of valves is called a *lymph angion*. The smooth musculature located in the medium layer of collectors contracts rhythmically, and has an autonomous contraction frequency of about 10–12 contractions per minute at rest (*lymphangiomotoricity*).

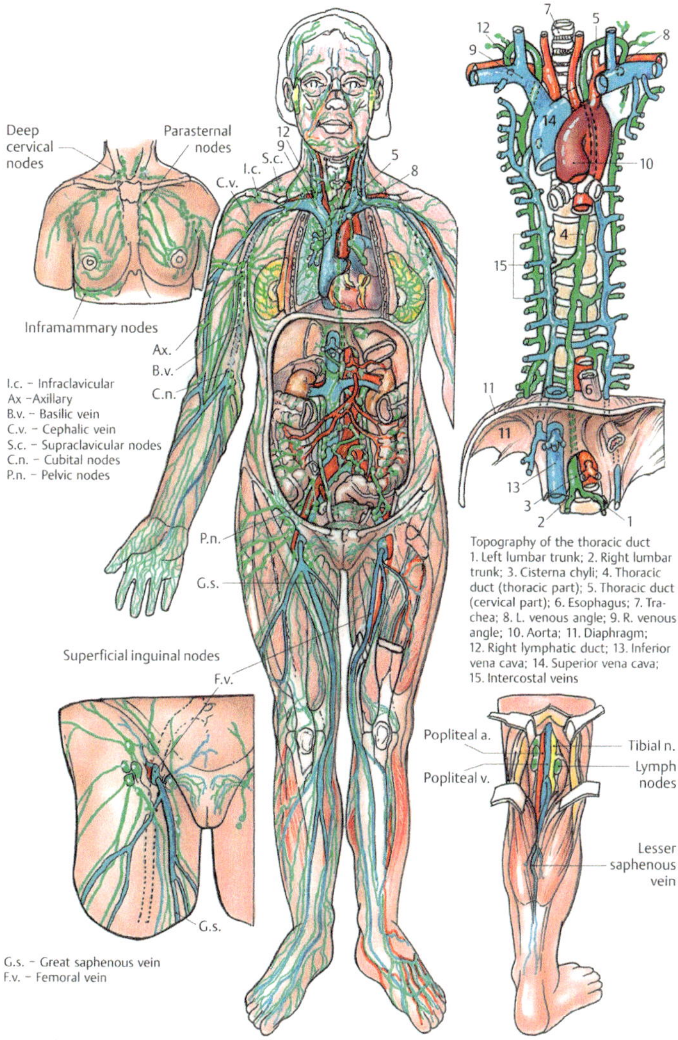

Fig. 1.3 Lymphatic system overview.
From Zuther J, Norton S Lymphedema Management, the Comprehensive Guide For Practitioners 4th ed. Thieme Publishers Stuttgart/New York (reprinted with permission)

Lymph collectors react to an increase in the volume of lymph fluid with an increase in the frequency of contractions of the smooth musculature within the angions. The increase in lymph fluid entering the lymph angion results in a stretch on the wall of the angion, which in turn results in an increase in lymphangiomotoricity.

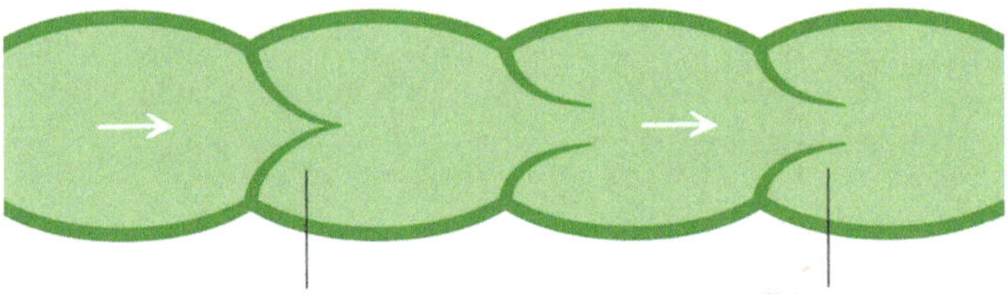

Fig. 1.4 Lymph collector with valves

The main function of lymph collectors is the drainage of lymph fluid from certain body areas, known as tributary or drainage areas. Most drainage areas of the superficial lymphatic system are subdivided into lymphatic territories.

Lymphatic territories consist of a number of collectors that are responsible for the drainage of the same body area; lymphatic territories are separated by lymphatic watersheds.

All collectors in a lymphatic territory transport lymph fluid towards the same group of lymph nodes, known as regional lymph nodes. In making their way toward the lymph nodes, collectors on the extremities run parallel to the watersheds, whereas collectors on the trunk tend to originate at the watersheds.

Trunks

Lymph fluid coming from the superficial and deep areas of the body are transported by collectors toward lymphatic trunks, which then carry the lymph back into the venous part of the blood circulatory system, where it enters into the right and left venous angles located on the lower end of the lateral neck behind the clavicle.

Lymphatic trunks exhibit the same structures as collectors with valves and a well developed smooth muscle structure in their walls, but are larger transport vessels.

The *right and left lumbar trunks* carry lymph fluid originating from the lower extremities, the lower body quadrants (below the naval line), and the external genitalia. Both lumbar trunks connect with the *cisterna chyli*, a 3-8 cm long sac-like reservoir located and behind the aorta and below the diaphragm. The *gastrointestinal trunk*, which brings lymph from the digestive system also connects with the cisterna chyli, which forms the beginning of the *thoracic duct*

Originating with the cisterna chyli, the thoracic duct represents the largest lymphatic trunk in the body, being between 36 and 45 cm long and about 0.5 cm wide. It passes through the diaphragm together with the aorta and empties in the majority of cases into the left venous angle, which is formed by the confluence of the left subclavian and internal jugular veins. Under normal conditions the majority of the lymph fluid collected throughout the body (about 2-3 liters per day) is returned to the blood via the thoracic duct in the left venous angle (Figs. 1.2, 1.3).

The remaining lymph fluid returns to the blood with the *right lymphatic duct*, which is formed by the confluence of the right subclavian and internal jugular veins (Fig 1.5).

Valves situated where the thoracic duct and the right lymphatic duct meets the venous system, prevent the flow of venous blood into the lymphatic system.

The *subclavian trunk*, located on both sides of the body, transports lymph fluid coming from the axillary lymph nodes, which are responsible for the filtration of lymph originating from the upper extremities, the upper quadrants (above the naval line) including the majority of the mammary gland, as well as the shoulder area.

Lymph fluid originating from portions of the head and neck area returns via the *jugular trunks*, which are located on both sides of the lower end of the neck, returning lymph back to the venous blood through the left and right venous angles.

The *supraclavicular trunks* transport lymph from the lymph nodes above the collar bone (supraclavicular lymph nodes), which filter lymph originating from the shoulder area and parts of the mammary gland. The right and left supraclavicular trunks empty into the blood via the left and right venous angles as well (Figs. 1.3, 1.5).

Comparison of Blood and Lymph Vessels

The circulatory system represents a closed system with the heart as its central motor, and blood vessels as the other structural elements. The main purpose of the blood vessels is the uninterrupted supply of all body tissues with nutrients and oxygenated blood, and the removal of metabolic waste and carbon dioxide from the tissue cells. The part of the circulatory system that delivers blood to and from the lungs is known as the pulmonary circulation, and the flow of blood throughout the rest of the body is administered by the systemic circulation.

The lymphatic system and its vessels do not form a closed circulatory system. It begins with small lymph capillaries in the body tissues, and continues with successively larger lymphatic vessels, collectors and trunks, which ultimately connect to the venous part of the blood circulatory system at the right and left venous angles. There is no central pump, lymph vessels produce their own propulsion system with a network of smooth musculature located in the walls of lymph collectors and trunks. Since the lymph vessels work according to the one-way principle and not as a closed circulatory system, it is more appropriate to speak of lymph transport rather than lymph circulation. While the flow of blood through the blood vessels is uninterrupted, the transport of lymph fluid through the lymph vessel system is interrupted by lymph nodes.

1.3 Lymph Fluid

Once the tissue fluid enters the lymphatic capillaries, it is called lymph. Lymph fluid is a clear and, except for the cloudy fluid found in lymph vessels draining the intestinal system.

Lymph fluid is composed of lymphatic loads, a term summarizing various substances that leave the tissue areas via the lymphatic system. Lymphatic loads include protein, water, cellular components and particles, and fat.

Protein

During the course of a day at least half of the proteins circulating in the blood will leave along the blood capillaries and travel into the tissue spaces; given this fact, the protein concentration in the tissues continues to remain lower than that of the blood. Proteins in the body tissues perform such important tasks as cell nutrition, immune defense, and blood coagulation. They are also responsible for the transport of fats, minerals, hormones, and waste products. Proteins also play a vital role in fluid balance.

Proteins are unable to re-enter the bloodstream via the blood capillaries; the return of the proteins circulating in the tissues back into the bloodstream is facilitated by the lymphatic system. Openings between the cells of lymph capillaries allow the large protein molecules to be absorbed.

The implications resulting from insufficient protein return in case of lymphedema will be discussed in the next chapter.

Water

A portion of the water leaving the blood capillary system by way of filtration comprises the lymphatic load of water. This remaining fraction is returned to the blood circulation via the thoracic duct, the right lymphatic duct, and the venous angles, and amounts to approximately 2–3 liters per day. However, considerably larger volumes of lymphatic load of water than the roughly 3 liters returned by the thoracic duct and the right lymphatic duct are produced throughout the body during the day. The remaining portion of water is absorbed by blood capillaries inside the lymph nodes.

The lymphatic load of water plays an essential role in the body's fluid management and serves as a solvent for other lymphatic loads.

Cells and Particles

White blood cells (lymphocytes) leave the blood capillaries into the tissues continuously and are picked up by the lymphatics. The circulation of lymphocytes back into the bloodstream plays an essential role in the immune response of the body.

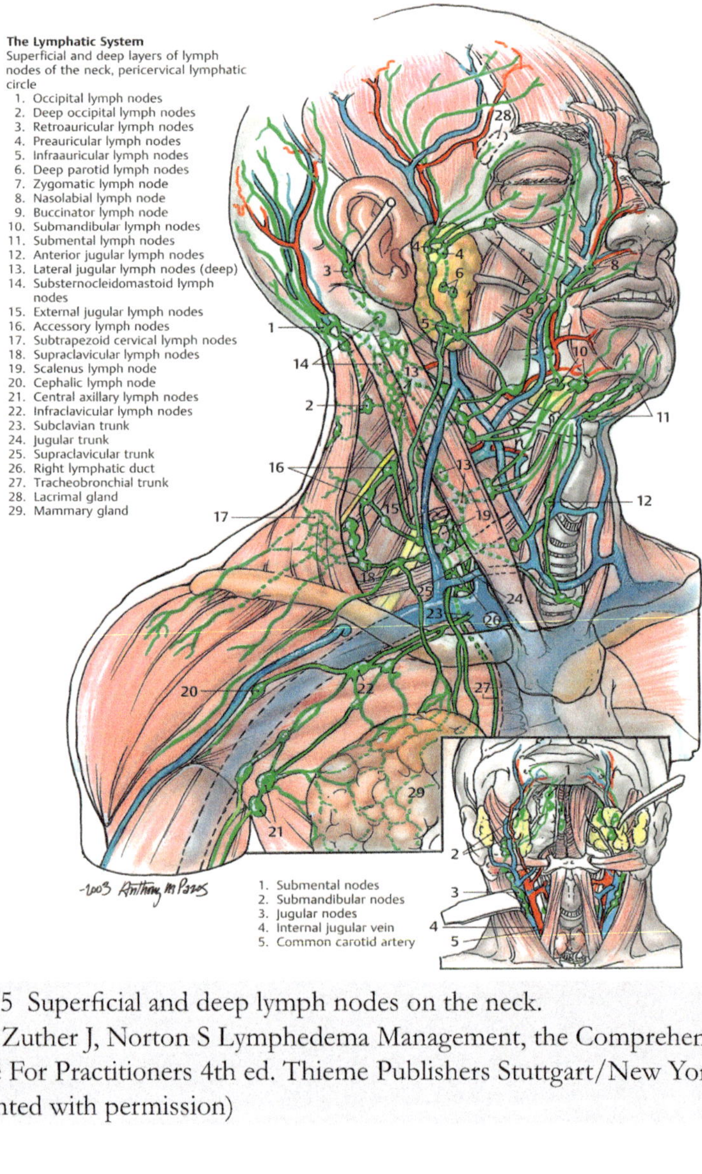

Fig. 1.5 Superficial and deep lymph nodes on the neck.
From Zuther J, Norton S Lymphedema Management, the Comprehensive Guide For Practitioners 4th ed. Thieme Publishers Stuttgart/New York (reprinted with permission)

Cancer cells use the lymphatic system to form metastases in lymph nodes and other tissues. Other cell fractions resulting from trauma or formation of new tissue, as well as bacteria and other particles entering the body by way of inhalation, digestion, or injury (dust, dirt, fungal spores, and other cellular components) are also absorbed by the lymphatic vessels and transported to the lymph nodes, where immune response mechanisms are activated.

Fatty Acids

The blood vessels of the small intestines are unable to absorb certain fat compounds and are picked up by the intestinal lymph vessels, also referred to in the literature as chylous vessels, which return fatty acids and fat compounds back to the bloodstream. Once fatty acids are part of the lymph, the normally transparent lymph fluid takes on a milky color.

1.4 Lymphatic Drainage of Body Areas

In the vast majority of cases lymphedema presents in the area of the skin and subcutis, affecting the superficial lymphatic network. The focus of the below text segment is on the superficial system and only occasionally comments on the deeper layers of the lymphatic system.

Head and Neck

The lymphatic vessels and lymph nodes in this area are divided into a superficial and deep system; the majority of lymph nodes responsible for the filtration of lymph fluid originating in the scalp and face area are arranged as a ring along the border of the head and neck, and are summarily referred to as the pericervical lymphatic circle (Fig 1.5).

Lymph nodes belonging to this group are the

- occipital lymph nodes (1-3 nodes), located at the lateral border of the trapezius muscle at the back of the head and collect lymph fluid from the posterior area of the scalp and the upper portion of the skin on the neck

- mastoid, or posterior auricular nodes (1-3), located behind the ear at the insertion of the sternocleidomastoid muscle. They collect lymph from the upper portion of the scalp, posterior ear and the skin of the neck
- pre-auricular and parotid lymph nodes (3-9), located directly in front of the ear and embedded in the fatty tissue surrounding the parotid gland. These nodes collect lymph from the temporal area of the scalp, forehead, anterior ear, upper eye lid and the lateral portion of the lower lid
- submandibular lymph nodes (3-6), located behind the mandible with the saliva gland, collecting lymph fluid from the cheeks, nose, upper eye lid and medial portion of the lower lid, chin and lateral portion of the lower lip.
- Submental lymph nodes (2-3), located in the fatty tissue above the mylohoid muscle behind the chin, responsible for the collection of lymph from the chin and central part of the lower lip.

The deep lymph nodes on the neck (cervical nodes; about 10-20) collect all the lymph fluid originating from the head and neck, either directly, or indirectly via the superficial cervical lymph nodes, the larynx, pharynx, trachea and thyroid gland, tongue, hard and soft palate, and tonsils.

The nodes are arranged into a vertical chain, which runs parallel and in close proximity to the internal jugular vein. The efferent vessels from this chain converge to form the right and left jugular trunks (Fig 1.5).

Supraclavicular lymph nodes (4-12) are part of this group and located behind the clavicle; these nodes filter fluid coming from the skin on the front of the neck, part of the mammary gland and lateral upper arm. The efferent vessels from this chain converge to form the right and left supraclavicular trunks, which connect to the venous angles (Figs. 1.3, 1.5).

Cervical lymph nodes are a common site of metastases for malignant tumors, most commonly from head and neck primary tumors. The proximity and possible connections of the supraclavicular trunk with the thoracic duct and other trunks terminating in the venous angle area explain why metastatic tumors from distant tumors, such as the mammary gland, lung, and esophagus, as well as from reproductive and intestinal organs, can be found in the supraclavicular lymph nodes.

Upper Extremity

The lymphatic system of the arm can be separated into a deep and superficial layer, and connections between these layers are present in both directions; in the hand area, connections from deep to superficial dominates. Axillary lymph nodes are the regional nodes for both layers.

The lymph collectors belonging to the deep layer generally follow the path of major deep blood vessels (ulnar, radial and brachial arteries and veins). These collectors are responsible for the filtration of lymph fluid originating from the muscles, tendons, joint capsules and periosteum.

Lymph collectors belonging to the superficial system of the upper extremity originate from the initial lymph vessels (capillaries) of the hand and travel up the arm accompanying the larger superficial veins.

Forearm: Collectors in this area are subdivided into the radial, ulnar, and median territories, or bundles. The median forearm territory is located on the frontal surface of the forearm. Collectors coming from the back of the hand continue along the forearm with the radial and ulnar forearm territories, which accompany the cephalic and basilic veins, respectively. The collectors of both bundles run around the forearm to converge with the median territory in the area in front of the elbow (antecubital), where they decrease in number (Fig. 1.6 a/b).

Cubital lymph nodes, located adjacent to the basilic vein provide additional filter stations for the collectors of the ulnar territory.

Upper Arm: The forearm collectors continue to travel to the axillary lymph node group along the medial upper arm territory, which is located between the biceps and the triceps muscles on the inner aspect of the upper arm. These collectors also transport lymph from the inner portion of the upper arm.

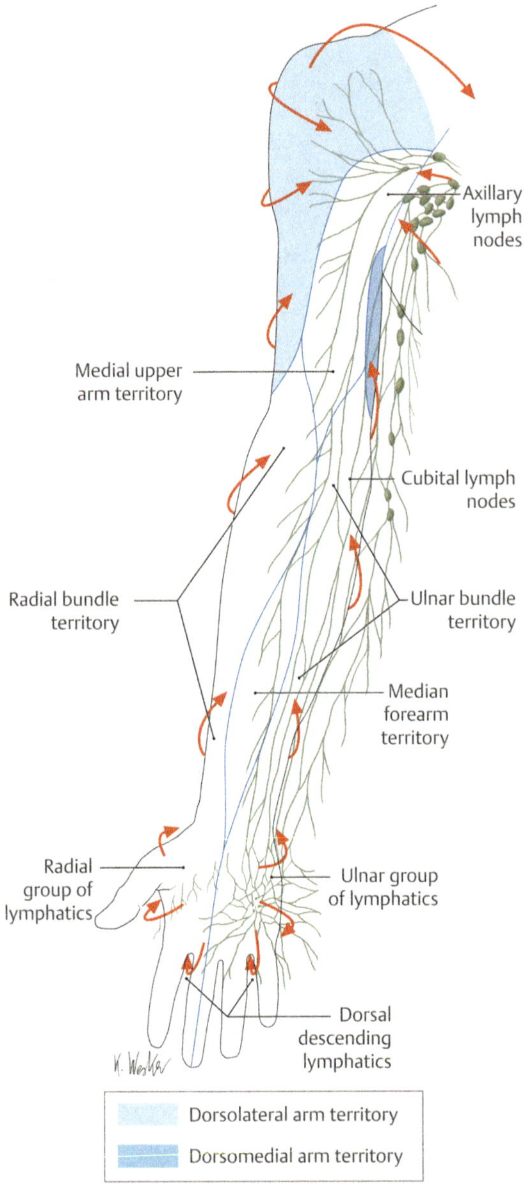

Fig. 1.6 (a) Superficial lymphatic system of the upper extremity frontal aspect

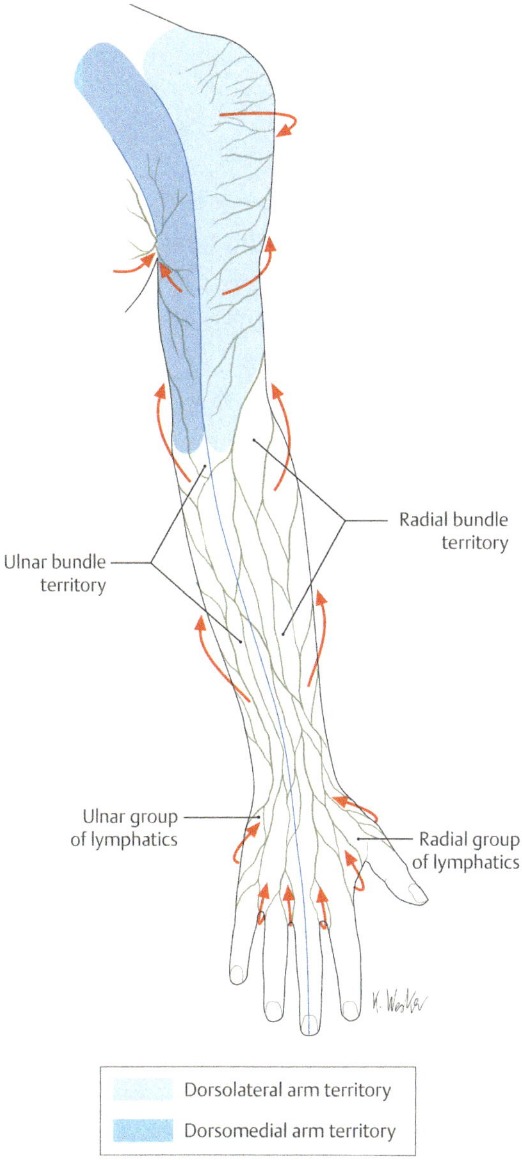

Fig. 1.6 (b) Superficial lymphatic system of the upper extremity posterior aspect.
From Wittlinger H Dr.Vodder's Manual Lymph Drainage. Thieme Stuttgart/ New York; 2001 (reprinted with permission

The lateral upper arm territory is responsible for the drainage of the skin on the outer aspect of the upper arm and shoulder. Its collectors drain partly into axillary and supraclavicular lymph nodes.

Axillary Lymph Nodes

Axillary lymph nodes are embedded in the fatty tissue of the underarm area located between the posterior border of the pectoralis, and the anterior border of the latissimus muscles; the number of nodes varies between 20 and 40. These nodes are responsible for filtering lymph fluid originating from the upper extremity, the majority of the mammary gland and the upper body quadrants (above the naval line) front and back, and are arranged into 5 groups (Figs. 1.5, 1.7):

- Lateral (infraclavicular) nodes are located in the anterior wall of the armpit. They collect lymph from the arm and drain into the central, and apical axillary nodes, and from there to deep cervical nodes.
- Posterior (subscapular) lymph nodes are located on the posterior wall of the armpit along the lower border of the subscapularis muscle. They collect lymph from the posterior wall of the upper body quadrant and drain into the central and apical axillary nodes.
- Central axillary lymph nodes reside in the center of the armpit and collect lymph from the anterior, posterior, and lateral groups, and drain to the apical axillary nodes.
- Apical nodes are located deep in the upper center of the axilla. They receive lymph from all of the groups mentioned above and the upper lateral mammary gland. The collectors leading away (efferent vessels) from the apical group converge to form the subclavian lymphatic trunk. On the left, the subclavian trunk drains directly into the thoracic duct, and on the right into the right venous angle via the right lymphatic duct.
- Anterior (pectoral) lymph nodes are arranged along the border of the pectoralis muscle. These nodes collect lymph from the breast, skin, and muscles of the anterior upper body quadrant (above the naval line) and drain into the central and apical nodes.

The axillary lymph nodes are of particular significance as these nodes are often present as the first site of metastases from breast cancer.

Upper Body Quadrants and Mammary Gland

Four quadrants or territories can be differentiated on the trunk. They are located above the naval line, also known as the horizontal watershed; both upper quadrants are further separated in the middle by a line running vertically in the front and back of the body, which is also known as the sagittal watershed. The lymph collectors of the upper quadrants are arranged like spokes on a wheel, with the origin emanating from the watersheds that outline these quadrants; The collectors follow in a fairly straight line toward the axillary nodes, which are the regional lymph nodes of this area.

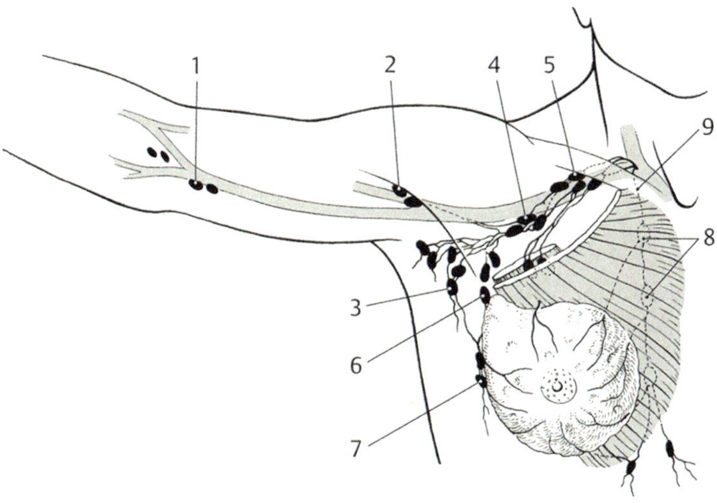

Fig. 1.7 Drainage of the mammary gland with axillary and parasternal lymph nodes. 1, cubital nodes; 2, lateral (infraclavicular) nodes; 3, posterior nodes; 4, central axillary nodes; 5, apical nodes; 6, anterior nodes; 7, paramammary nodes; 8, parasternal nodes (internal mammary nodes); 9, parasternal trunk.
From Zuther J, Norton S Lymphedema Management, the Comprehensive Guide For Practitioners 4th ed. Thieme Publishers Stuttgart/New York (reprinted with permission)

The lymph collectors of the mammary gland drain into two groups of lymph nodes (Fig. 1.7). The dominant pathway is represented by collectors draining the lateral breast quadrants, which drain around 75% of the mammary gland; these collectors terminate in the axillary lymph nodes. The medial quadrants of the breast is drained by collectors running towards the parasternal (internal mammary nodes) lymph nodes, which are located next to the sternum in the intercostal spaces.

From there the lymph fluid is transported via the parasternal trunk towards the left and right venous angles.

Lower Extremity

As with the arm, the lymph vessels on the lower extremity are divided into a superficial and deep system. The deep lymphatic layer drains muscles, tendons, ligaments, and joints. The deep lymph collectors below the knee contain three sets of collectors, the anterior and posterior tibial and the peroneal collectors, which accompany the corresponding blood vessels. All three transport the lymph to the deep popliteal lymph nodes (4-6), which are embedded in the fat contained in the back of the knee (popliteal fossa). From there, collectors follow the femoral artery and terminate in the deep inguinal lymph nodes.

The deep collectors on the thigh tend to follow the deep femoral artery and run toward the deep inguinal lymph nodes. Collectors of the buttock area follow the gluteal artery and transport the lymph fluid to the pelvic lymph nodes.

Lymph collectors belonging to the superficial system of the lower extremity originate from the initial lymph vessels (capillaries) of the foot and travel up the leg accompanying the larger superficial veins.

Foot: The meshes of the lymph capillaries are finer on the sole of the foot and toes. Collectors on the back of the foot drain most of the sole, the toes, and the medial ankle area, and pass the ankle on the front and medial side to continue as part of the *ventromedial territory* on the lower leg. Collectors draining the lateral ankle and the lateral border of the foot, including portions of the lateral sole, continue as collectors belonging to the *posterolateral territory* on the leg towards the popliteal lymph nodes in the back of the knee (Figs. 1.8 a/b).

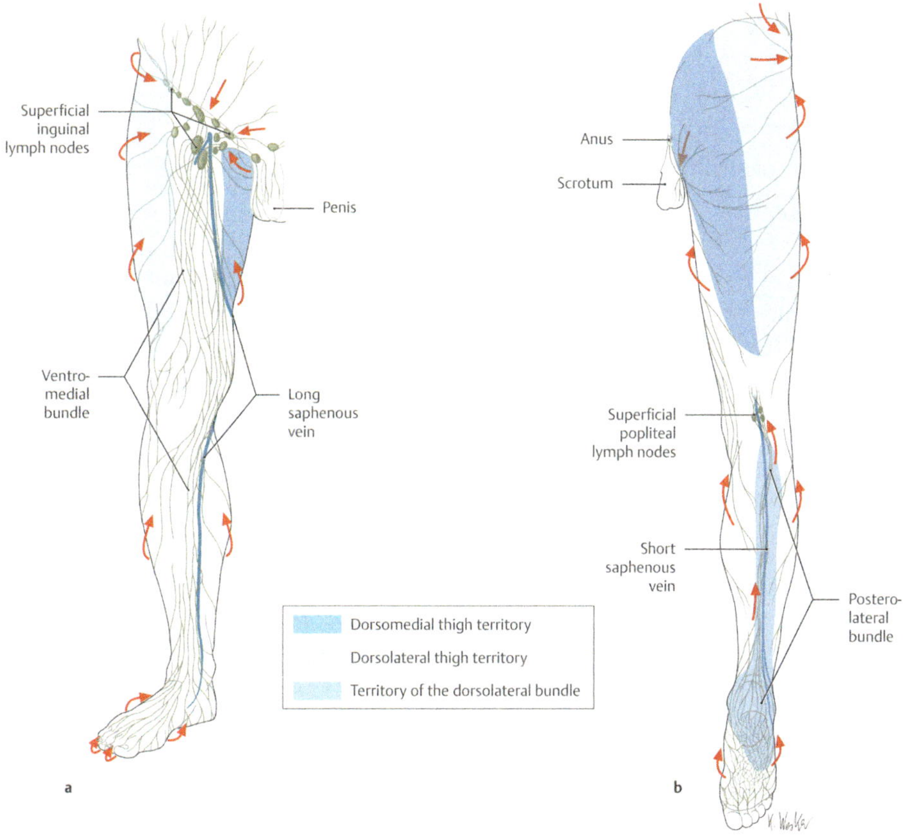

Fig. 1.8 a (anterior leg) b (posterior leg) Superficial lymphatic system and territories of the lower extremity and the adjacent trunk quadrant. Arrows indicate the drainage direction. From Wittlinger H Dr.Vodder's Manual Lymph Drainage. Thieme Stuttgart/New York; 2001 (reprinted with permission)

Lower Leg and Knee: Two territories can be differentiated on the lower leg. The *ventromedial territory* drains most of the foot as a continuation of the collectors coming from the back of the foot and the medial ankle, as well as the skin of the lower leg, except an area of skin in the middle of the calf. Collectors of the ventromedial group are larger and more numerous than those of the posterolateral territory. Collectors of the posterolateral group begin on the lateral and posterior border of the foot, drain the portion of skin located in the middle of the calf, and follow the small saphenous vein to the superficial popliteal lymph nodes. From the superficial popliteal lymph nodes, the lymph fluid continues to the deep popliteal lymph nodes and continue to follow deep lymph collectors to the deep inguinal lymph nodes.

Collectors of the ventromedial territory run up the leg with the great saphenous vein and pass with it behind the medial knee to the thigh. The vessels decrease in number below the medial knee to an average of 4–6 collectors (from 5–10 on the lower leg).

Thigh: The collectors of the ventromedial territory continue to follow the great saphenous vein to the superficial inguinal lymph nodes. The *dorsolateral thigh territory* drains the skin of the lateral thigh and the lateral buttock area. The *dorsomedial thigh territory* is responsible for the medial thigh, the medial buttock, and the perineum.

Inguinal Lymph Nodes

The inguinal lymph nodes can be subdivided into two groups, the superficial inguinal lymph nodes (6-12 nodes) and the deep inguinal nodes (1-3 nodes).

The superficial group is embedded in the fatty tissue in the groin around the great saphenous vein and is found in the upper part of the medial femoral triangle, which is outlined by the inguinal ligament, the sartorius muscle, and the adductor muscles of the thigh. The superficial nodes can be further divided into two groups, the nodes belonging to the horizontal group are arranged as a chain, which is located immediately below the inguinal ligament. The nodes arranged around the medial femoral vein belong to the vertical group (Figs. 1.8 a, 1.9).

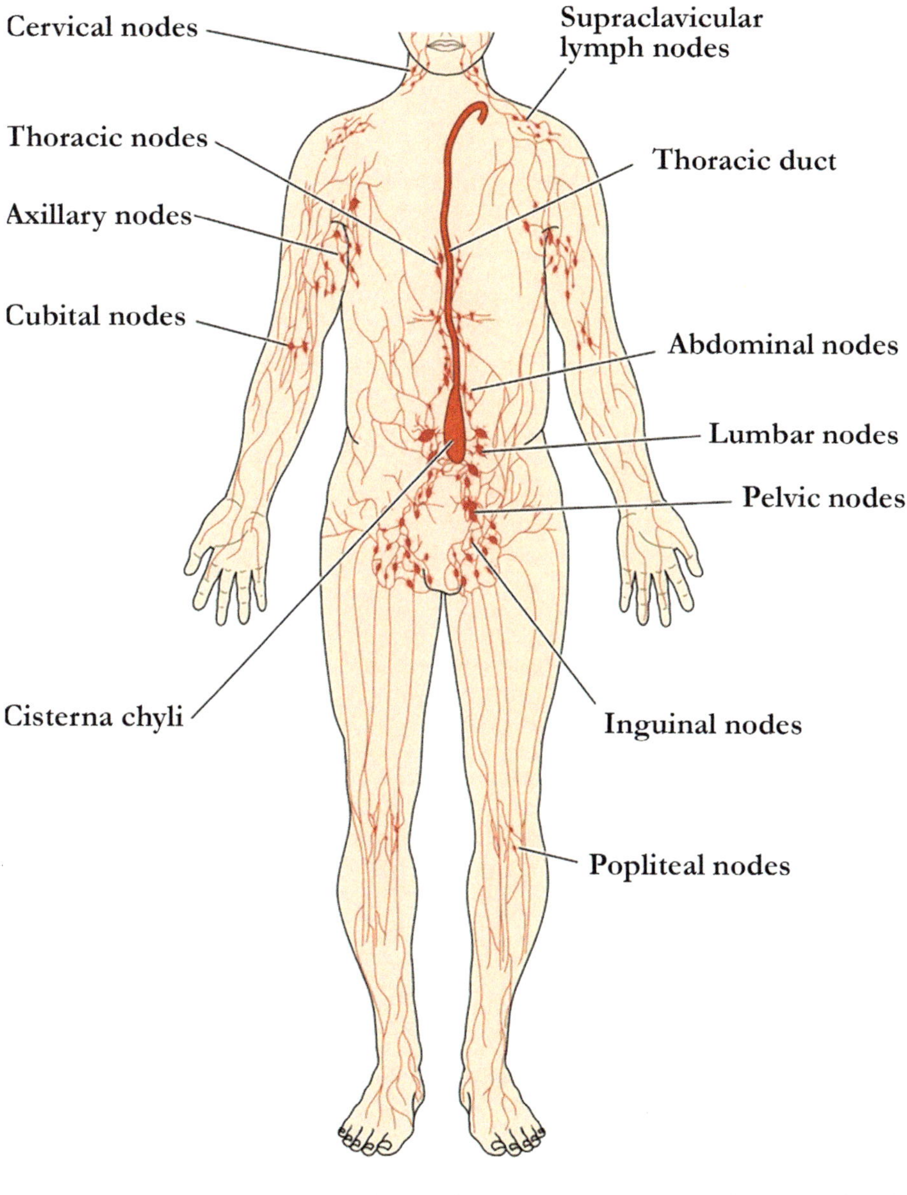

Fig 1.9 Lymph node groups

The horizontal group receives lymph fluid from the skin tissue of the penis, scrotum, lower part of the vagina, perineum, anus, buttock, and anterior and posterior lower body quadrants (below the naval line). The vertical group is mainly responsible for the drainage and filtration of lymph coming from the superficial lymphatic collectors of the lower extremity; they also receive some of the lymph collectors that drain the skin of the penis, scrotum, vagina, perineum, and buttock area.

From the inguinal lymph nodes, the lymph continues to be transported by collectors that perforate the body's fascia below the inguinal ligament, following the pelvic artery to connect with the pelvic lymph nodes (Fig. 1.9). From there the lymph fluid continues to pass through the lumbar lymph nodes (located along the lumbar vertebrae) and the lumbar trunks to reach the cisterna chyli and the thoracic duct (Figs. 1.3, 1.9).

The deep inguinal nodes are situated below the body fascia in the medial femoral triangle and receive the lymph transported by the deep lymph collectors accompanying the femoral artery, lymph fluid from the glans and corpus penis, and the outer layer of the clitoris. Lymph fluid previously filtered by the superficial inguinal lymph nodes also passes through the deep group.

Lower Body Quadrants

As with the upper body quadrants, the anterior and posterior lower quadrants are outlined by the horizontal and sagittal watersheds, the lower quadrants are located below the naval line (horizontal watershed). The lymph collectors of the lower quadrants are arranged like spokes on a wheel, with the origin emanating from the watersheds that outline these quadrants. The collectors follow in a fairly straight line toward the superficial inguinal nodes, which are the regional lymph nodes of this area.

References

(1) Louveau, A. et al. Structural and functional features of central nervous system lymphatic vessels. Nature. 2015 523(7560): 337- 341. doi:10.1038/nature14432.Published online June 1 2015

(2) Aspelund, A. et al. A dural lymphatic vascular system that drains brain interstitial fluid and macromolecules. Exp. Med., 2015; 212(7):991–999

(3) Bradstreet JJ, Pacini S, Ruggiero M. A New Methodology of Viewing Extra-Axial Fluid and Cortical Abnormalities in Children with Autism via Transcranial Ultrasonography. Front Hum Neurosci 2014; 15(7): 934. doi: 3389/fnhum.2013.00934

(4) Louveau A, Herz J, Alme MN, et al. CNS lymphatic drainage and neuroinflammation are regulated by meningeal lymphatic vasculature.

Nat Neurosci 2018; 21: 1380-1391. doi: 10.1038/s41593-018-0227-9

(5) Matarazzo EB. Treatment of late onset autism as a consequence of probable autoimmune processes related to chronic bacterial infection. World J Biol Psychiatry 2002; 3(3): 162-166.

6) Nicola Antonucci, Stefania Pacini and Marco Ruggiero, Biomedical Centre for Autism Research and Treatment, Bari, Italy and Silver Spring Sagl, Arzo-Mendrisio, Switzerland. Manual Lymphatic Drainage in Autism Treatment; Madridge J Immunol Vol.3, Issue 1

2.0 Lymphedema

The term "swelling" is used to describe an enlargement of a body part and can be used to describe edema, as well as lymphedema. While the initial causes for the formation of the swelling are different, both involve the accumulation of fluid in the soft tissues of the skin due to some form of insufficiency of the lymphatic system. However, edema and lymphedema are clearly not the same and require different treatment approaches.

2.1 Definition and Incidence

Lymphedema is a progressive and chronic condition with an abnormal build-up of protein-rich fluid in the tissues, which is caused by a disruption or obstruction of normally functioning lymph vessels or lymph nodes in certain parts of the body. It develops if the transport capacity of the lymphatic system has fallen below the normal amount of lymph fluid the lymphatic system is able transport. This can be caused by damage to, or a developmental abnormality of the lymphatic system.

The transport capacity of the lymphatic system is the maximum amount of fluid the lymphatic system can handle. In a healthy lymphatic system, the transport capacity exceeds the normal amount of lymph fluid by a factor of almost 10, which allows the lymphatic system to react to an increased volume of water and proteins by increasing its activity and cope with the additional volume.

Lymphedema generally presents in the arms and legs; however, other parts of the body, such as trunk, abdomen, head and neck, external genitalia, and internal organs can be affected as well. The onset of lymphedema can be gradual in some patients and sudden in others. Most patients develop lymphedema following surgery and/or radiation therapy for various cancers, in which case it is referred to as secondary lymphedema. Primary lymphedema develops without obvious cause at different stages in life due to abnormalities in the development of the lymphatic system.

Lymphedema is a very common condition, affecting 140-250 million people worldwide, and at least three million Americans. The most common cause for lymphedema in developing countries is filariasis, which is a parasitic infestation of the lymphatic system, accounting for millions of cases (see later in this chapter).

Resulting from a general lack of literature on the incidence of primary and secondary lymphedema, and the variety of techniques and definitions used in studies that evaluate this condition, there is no reliable data on the incidence of lymphedema.

Most data is available on the incidence of breast cancer, which is the most common cause for secondary lymphedema affecting the upper extremities and trunkal area. Next to skin cancer, breast cancer is the most common form of cancer in women.

While the overall cancer-related incidence rate of secondary lymphedema in the US is 15%, the long-term breast cancer treatment related incidence rate of secondary lymphedema is about 50%. In other words, half of women will develop some degree of lymphedema following breast cancer surgery within 20 years after treatment[(1)].

To put that in perspective, generally it can be said that one out of eight women in the US will develop breast cancer during the course of their lives. Statistics available from the Centers of Disease Control and Prevention (CDC) and the American Cancer Society indicate that around 270,000 new cases of breast cancer in females and 2700 cases in males are diagnosed annually in the US, with rising incidence[(2)].

Incidence data of lower extremity lymphedema resulting from malformations, or damage to the lymphatic system secondary to surgical procedures for cancers (gynecological, prostate, colorectal, pancreatic, testicular, skin cancer) or other conditions, such as lymphedema developing as a result of chronic venous insufficiencies or lipedema is even less available.

Lower extremity lymphedema is often under-recognized and, as a result, under-served as a patient group.

Head and neck lymphedema (HNL) is a common side effect of head and neck cancer treatment. It has been estimated that more than 50% of treated head and neck cancer patients will develop some degree of lymphedema affecting the head and neck.

2.2 Insufficiencies of the Lymphatic System

A lymphatic insufficiency is present if the transport capacity of the lymphatic system is smaller than the volume of lymphatic fluid; there are three forms of insufficiency, which can result in either edema or lymphedema: dynamic, mechanical, or combined insufficiency.

Dynamic Insufficiency

This is the most common insufficiency, also known as high-volume insufficiency. In this case, the volume of water (sometimes of protein and water) exceeds the transport capacity of the healthy lymphatic system, which will result in *edema.* Edema is a swelling caused by the accumulation of abnormally large amounts of fluid in the tissue spaces of the body, which is visible and/or palpable (pitting). It is a symptom rather than a disease or disorder, and may be caused by cardiac insufficiency, immobility, chronic venous insufficiency (stage 1 and 2), pregnancy, and other factors.

Prolonged dynamic insufficiency can cause secondary damage to the lymphatic system. The constant overload causes the lymph collectors to work at their transport capacity over extended periods of time, possibly resulting in damage to the structure of the walls and valves of lymph collectors. Secondary damage to the lymph collectors could cause a reduction in their transport capacity, which could further exacerbate the situation.

To avoid secondary damage to the lymphatic system and the tissues, it is imperative to reduce the amount of swelling as soon as possible. In localized edema, this can be achieved by elevation, exercise, and compression, as long as the overload is not caused by cardiac insufficiency, in which case compression therapy is contraindicated. In some instances, diuretics may be prescribed to reduce the edema.

Mechanical Insufficiency

This form, also known as low-volume insufficiency, is caused by a reduction in the transport capacity of the lymphatic system secondary to surgery, radiation, trauma, or inflammation involving the lymphatic system. The impairment is so severe that the lymphatic system is unable to perform one of its basic functions, which is the removal of water and protein from the tissues, or to respond to an increase in the lymphatic load of water and protein. This will result in high-protein edema or *lymphedema.*

Lymphedema, if left untreated, will lead to serious consequences. The stagnation of water, protein, and other waste products in the tissues may cause tissue damage, such as fibrosis, and leads to a high susceptibility to infections (cellulitis).

Combined Insufficiency

In this case, the transport capacity of the lymphatic system is below its normal level, and in addition to this, the amount of lymph fluid is elevated. The maximum degree of this insufficiency is reached if the transport capacity is reduced below the level of normal lymphatic fluid (mechanical insufficiency), and simultaneously the volume of lymph fluid is greater than the transport capacity of a healthy lymphatic system (dynamic insufficiency). The combination of these insufficiencies may lead to severe tissue damage (wounds) and chronic inflammation in the affected areas.

2.3 Primary Lymphedema

Primary lymphedema is far less common than the secondary form; it has been estimated to affect 1 in 100,000 people worldwide[3], most commonly female patients with a ratio of one male to three females. In most cases of primary lymphedema cases, the lower extremities are affected.

The formation of primary lymphedema is caused by developmental abnormality, affecting the structure and function of the lymphatic system directly. Most common forms of these malformations are *hypoplasia* or *hyperplasia* involving lymph vessels and/or lymph nodes.

Hypoplasia is the most common malformation, and refers to an incomplete development; the number of lymph vessels and/or nodes in this case is reduced, or the size of these lymphatic structures is smaller than normal.

Hyperplasia is generally associated with a structural malformation of lymph vessels and/or nodes, which is also known as lymphangiectasia, or megalymphatics. Enlargement (dilation) of lymph vessels in this case may result in a malfunction of valves located within the lymph collectors, compromising the flow of lymphatic fluid. This can be compared to dilated veins and insufficient valves caused by chronic venous insufficiencies (CVI), causing pooling, or stagnation of venous blood in the veins.

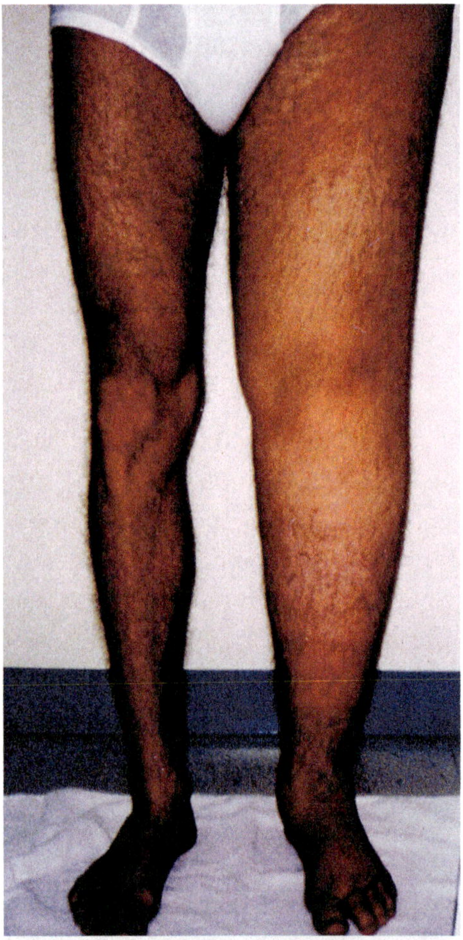

Fig. 2.1 Primary lymphedema of the left leg. From Zuther J, Norton S Lymphedema Management, the Comprehensive Guide For Practitioners 4th ed. Thieme Publishers Stuttgart/New York (reprinted with permission)

Lymphatic aplasia is rare and describes the absence or poor development of single lymph vessels and/or nodes.

The developmental abnormalities of the lymphatic system in primary lymphedema are inherited, which means it can pass from generation to generation. Several genes (VEGFR3, FOXC2, SOX18, ANGPT2, others) can be involved in the development of the lymphatic system[4] and mutations of any of these genes may cause lymphedema. However, only one of these genes is typically responsible for the lymphatic malformation in a particular family. Inherited lymphedema presents in an autosomal dominant pattern, which means that the gene in question is located on one of the numbered, or non-sex chromosomes, with incomplete penetrance and variable expression.

Primary lymphedema can also be associated with a known syndrome (Turner, Noonan, Hennekam, and others).

Except for genes on the sex chromosomes, both males and females have two copies of each gene. If only one altered copy of a gene (mutation) causes a malformation, the condition will be inherited in what is called a dominant pattern, which essentially means that children of parents with primary lymphedema have a 50% chance of inheriting the defective gene. This, however, does not explain why primary lymphedema is more common in female offspring; further studies to shed more light on this phenomenon are necessary.

In genetics the strength of a gene is described as penetrance; a strong penetrance is present if all children who inherit the abnormal gene develop primary lymphedema. If only a limited number of children who inherit the abnormal gene develop the condition, the penetrance is described as inconsistent or variable. This is the case with the lymphedema gene; not all children who inherit the mutation will show evidence of lymphedema. In many cases of primary lymphedema it can be established that the condition skipped one or more generations.

Variable expression indicates that the swelling may affect the left leg of one family member, another family member's right foot, and yet another family member may have both legs involved.

In addition, the age of presentation can also be variable. Although the abnormalities in the development of the lymphatic system are present at birth, lymphedema may develop at any point later in life, most often during puberty or pregnancy with a peak in the onset between the ages 10 and 25. However, primary lymphedema may not visibly develop at all as long as the genetically compromised lymphatic system is sufficient enough to manage its workload.

Primary lymphedema can be classified by the age of the patient at the onset of the swelling. *Congenital (pediatric) lymphedema* is present at birth or within the first two years of life and accounts for 10-25% of all cases of primary lymphedema. Boys typically are affected at birth, and girls most often present with lymphedema during adolescence[5]. A subgroup of patients with congenital lymphedema has a familial pattern of inheritance, which is known as Milroy's disease (VEGFR3 mutation).

The most common form of primary lymphedema is termed *lymphedema praecox,* also known as Meige's disease (no known gene mutation); by definition, it becomes clinically evident after birth and before age 35. This condition accounts for 65-80% of all primary lymphedema cases and most often arises during puberty or pregnancy.

A relatively rare form of primary lymphedema is when the first signs of swelling appear after 35 years of age; this condition is called *lymphedema tarda.*

Recent developments in research indicate that drugs are beginning to become available to oppose or correct the effects of gene mutations[6,7].

2.4 Secondary Lymphedema

Secondary lymphedema results from an identifiable damage leading to disruption or obstruction of normally functioning lymph vessels and/or lymph nodes and may present in the extremities, trunk, abdomen, head and neck and external genitalia.

The highest incidence of secondary lymphedema in the United States is observed following surgery and radiation for malignancies, particularly among those individuals affected by breast cancer. Other surgeries, to include treatment of melanoma, cancer affecting the genitourinary and gynecologic systems, cancers in the head and neck region, or soft tissue malignancies, generally include the removal of lymph nodes with subsequent disruption of lymphatic pathways, may also cause the onset of secondary lymphedema.

All women are at risk for developing breast cancer; males are also affected at a ratio of one male to 100 females. With increasing age, the greater a woman's chance of developing breast cancer with most cancer cases occurring in women over 50 years of age. While breast cancer is less common at a young age, younger women tend to have more aggressive breast cancers than older women, which may explain why survival rates are lower among younger women. Incidence also varies within ethnic groups and geographical location within the US.

Attributable to increasing cancer rates, secondary lymphedema is becoming more common, affecting 1 in 1,000 individuals; 24–49% of cancer patients develop secondary lymphedema following cancer treatment[8]. The incidence rate is likely underestimated because lymphedema remains under-recognized and under-diagnosed to this day.

Any type of surgery, specifically procedures that require the removal of lymph nodes, can cause the onset of lymphedema. Surgical procedures in cancer therapy, such as breast conserving (lumpectomy) or more extensive breast surgery (mastectomy) commonly include the removal (dissection) of lymph nodes, with subsequent damage to lymph vessels.

Many individuals receive radiation therapy following the surgical procedure, which may further damage the lymphatic system. Radiation therapy, specifically if combined with the surgical removal of lymph nodes, can cause scarring in soft tissue and inflammation of lymph nodes and lymph vessels, which may also contribute to the development of secondary lymphedema. The goal of these procedures is to eliminate the cancer cells and to save the patient's life. However, a side effect in lymph node removal and/or radiation is the disruption in the transport of lymphatic fluid.

When the vessels are damaged, the flow of lymphatic fluid is compromised, and if the remaining lymph vessels that are unaffected by the surgery are not able to compensate for the damaged vessels, lymphatic fluid builds up in the tissues. This accumulation of lymphatic fluid results in abnormal swelling, most commonly affecting the upper and lower extremities; other parts of the body may be affected as well.

Less common causes for secondary lymphedema include surgeries other than for the treatment of malignancies, or trauma disrupting the flow of lymph. Tumors growing in the soft tissues can become large enough to cause a physical block on lymphatic structures subsequently obstructing the normal flow of lymph.

Secondary cases of lymphedema may occur immediately following the surgical procedure and/or radiation, within a few months, a couple of years, or twenty years or more after treatment. The average time of onset is between 14 and 24 months post-surgically, with an increased number of cases over time. Some individuals may never experience any symptoms; however, the risk of development of secondary lymphedema lasts a lifetime.

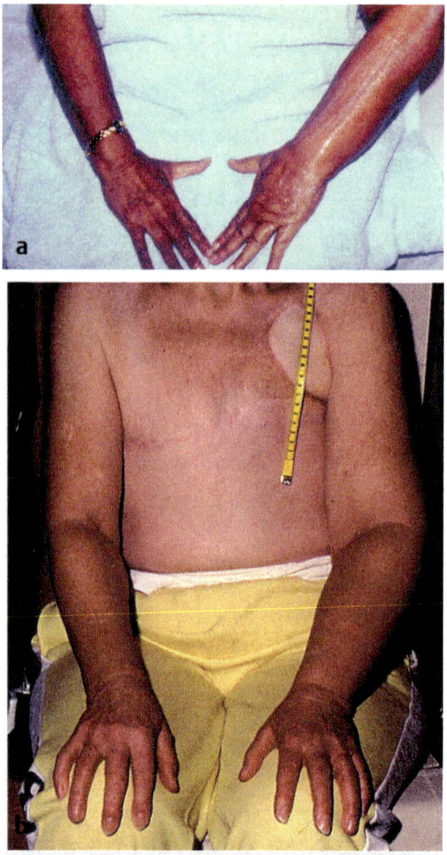

Fig. 2.2 (a) Sec. lymphedema left arm. (b) Sec. lymphedema left arm following bilateral mastectomy. From Zuther J, Norton S Lymphedema Management, 4th ed. Thieme Publishers Stuttgart /New York (reprinted with permission)

There is no consistency in the data on the incidence of lymphedema, and most statistics that are available are those on breast cancer related lymphedema (BCRL) affecting the upper extremities.

A study, which was published in 2001[1], followed 263 patients after mastectomy and complete axillary dissection. At 20 years after treatment, 49% reported lymphedema; of those, 77% noted onset within three years after surgery, and the remaining women developed lymphedema in the arm at a rate of almost 1% per year.

Patient education about the possibility of developing secondary lymphedema, discussion of the risk factors and risk reduction practices, combined with appropriate surveillance and prompt reporting of symptoms following cancer treatment, can limit the incidence and progression of secondary lymphedema.

In a study[9] including patients who received treatment for breast cancer, it was determined that patients who received information about the possible onset of secondary lymphedema demonstrated significantly reduced symptoms when compared with patients who did not receive this information. Women who received information about lymphedema were significantly less likely to report heaviness in the extremity, arm swelling, impaired shoulder mobility, and breast swelling.

Early treatment of secondary lymphedema by a qualified therapist is of paramount importance to limit progression of the swelling and to avoid complications often associated with untreated or incorrectly treated lymphedema.

Lymphedema Affecting the Breast and Trunk

Lymphedema affecting the chest, breast and posterior thorax, also known as trunkal lymphedema, is a common problem following breast cancer surgery, but is often difficult to diagnose, especially if the patient does not also present with lymphedema of the arm, or it may be dismissed as a side-effect of breast cancer surgery, which will resolve by itself over time.

While trunkal lymphedema is often not reported, poorly documented, and available studies are not easy to compare, the literature suggests an incidence of up to 70% of lymphedema affecting the trunk and/or breast following breast cancer treatment[15].

Given the fact that the breast, anterior and posterior thorax and the upper extremity share the axillary nodes as regional lymph nodes, it is predictable that disruption of lymphatic drainage pathways by partial or complete removal of axillary lymph nodes, with or without radiation therapy, can cause the onset of swelling in the chest wall and breast on the same side. The swelling can either be subtle or obvious in presentation and may be present with or without swelling in the arm.

The disruption of the natural lymphatic drainage pattern is further complicated by scars on the upper trunk wall following lumpectomy, mastectomy, and reconstructive breast surgery, biopsies or drain sites. Fibrotic tissues in the chest wall or armpit following radiation treatments may further inhibit sufficient lymphatic drainage.

Certain breast reconstructive procedures, such as the TRAM-flap reconstruction also disrupt lymphatic drainage in the abdominal area, which may cause the onset of additional swelling in the lower trunkal (abdominal) area.

Like lymphedema in the extremities, swelling affecting the breast, chest and posterior thorax is typically asymmetrical in appearance if compared with the other side. However, there are often other symptoms present prior to the onset of visible swelling, which may include altered sensation (numbness, tingling, diffuse fullness and pressure, heat), pain and decreased shoulder mobility. Once lymphedema is visibly present, the swelling may include the entire thorax wall, or may be localized to the armpit, the scapula, the area over the clavicle or around mastectomy/lumpectomy scar lines, around the reconstructed breast or implants, or it may be limited to the breast tissue.

The breast in patients who underwent lumpectomy or reconstructive surgery may be larger and heavier, or the shape and height of the breast tissue may change due to fibrotic tissue, resulting in added psychological distress due to problems involving clothing, bra fit and body image issues.

Post-operative swelling following breast cancer surgery is to be expected and generally lasts up to about three months; it appears almost immediately following surgery and places additional stress on the lymphatic system by contributing to the lymphatic workload. The difference between "normal" post-operative edema and lymphedema is its perseverance following the completion of treatment, and the presence of changes in tissue texture, such as lymphostatic fibrosis.

While several methods are available to assess trunkal and breast edema (skin fold calipers, MRI, CT), subjective examination of the anterior and posterior aspect of the thorax and breast focused on the observation of signs of swelling (asymmetry, bra strap and seam indentations, orange peel phenomenon, changes in skin color), palpation of the tissue texture and comparison of skin folds between the affected and non-affected side, remain the most practical means for assessment of lymphedema affecting the trunk. Serial photographs depicting the anterior and posterior view are helpful tools in assessing changes before and after treatment[10].

Lymphatic Filariasis

Lymphatic Filariasis, which is commonly known as elephantiasis, is a neglected, painful and disfiguring disease endemic to developing countries, and the leading cause for lymphedema in the world.

Lymphatic Filariasis has been identified by the World Health Organization (WHO) as a leading cause for permanent disability in the world; it is native to more than 80 regions in Africa, India, Southeast Asia, and South America, as well as in the Pacific islands and the Caribbean. According to the WHO, 863 million individuals in 47 countries remain threatened by lymphatic filariasis, and 51 million people were infected as of 2018, which represents a 74% decline since the WHO's start of a global program to eliminate the disease in 2000.

Filariasis is caused by three types of round parasitic filarial roundworms with Wucheria bancrofti being the most common type, responsible for 90% of infections. The other types are Brugia malayi and Brugia timori.

Lymphatic Filariasis is transmitted to humans by mosquitoes that carry infection-stage larvae; during the transmission, the larvae enter the body and are deposited in the individuals' skin; from there the parasitic larvae migrate to the lymphatic system, where over a period of 6-12 months they develop into adult worms and mate, thus continuing the cycle of transmission. Adult worms live for a period of about 4-6 years; male worms can grow 3-4 centimeters in length, whereas females can reach 8-10 centimeters.

Lymphatic Filariasis may present asymptomatic, with no external signs of disfigurement or infection but sub-clinical lymphatic damage, acute (infections, fever, swelling), or chronic.

The chronic stage includes lymphedema, which can grow to monstrous proportions and may affect the extremities (most often the legs), breasts and the external genitalia (labia, scrotum and penis) causing pain, disability and sexual dysfunction. Filarial worms inside the human lymphatic system cause dilation and damage to the lymphatics, restricting the normal flow of lymph, causing swelling, fibrosis and infections to lymph vessels and nodes (lymphangitis, lymphadenitis).

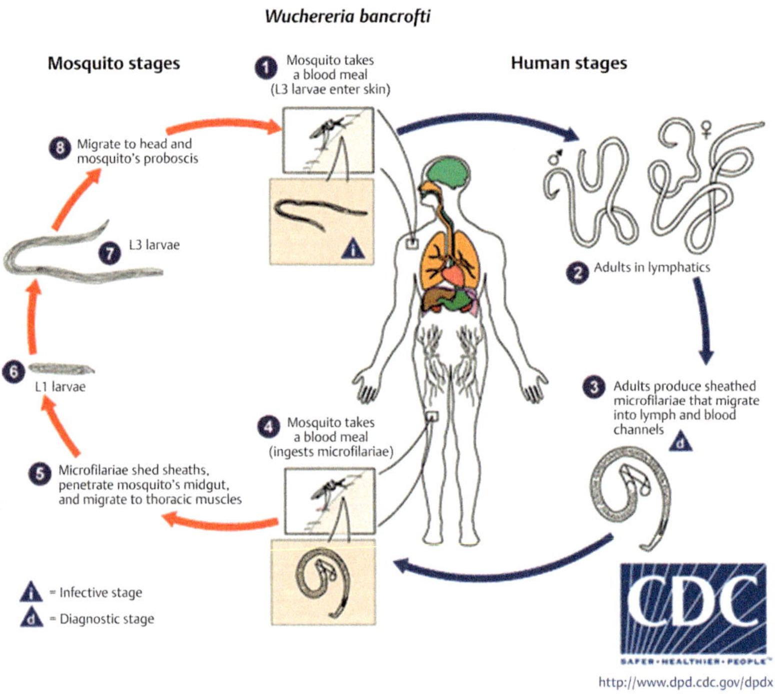

Fig. 2.3 Life cycle of Wucheria bancrofti. From Zuther J, Norton S Lymphedema Management, 4th ed. Thieme Publishers Stuttgart /New York (reprinted with permission)

Lymphatic Filariasis is typically diagnosed by blood tests detecting the presence of microfilariae in the blood, as well as antigen detection tests.

The WHO launched a global program to eliminate lymphatic filariasis (GPELF) in 2000, which aims to stop the spread of infections and to alleviate the suffering caused by this condition by large-scale administration of preventative chemotherapy. This involves the administration of an annual dose of medicines to the entire at-risk population; the primary drugs used are diethylcarbamazine citrate (DEC), albendazole and ivermectin, which effectively reduce circulating microfilariae, thus interrupting the transmission cycle. Research shows that the administration of a combination of these three drugs can safely clear microfilariae from the circulating blood in infected individuals within a week.

Filariasis is rare in the US but may be contracted by visiting countries where this disease is common. Foreigners visiting endemic countries are rarely infected; however, as a preventative measure mosquito bites should be avoided by sleeping under a mosquito net, using insect repellents, wearing long-sleeved shirts and long pants and refrain from being outside between dusk and dawn, when mosquitoes are most active.

Pediatric Lymphedema

When we think of lymphedema, we usually picture an adult; however, this is not always the case. Every year, children are being diagnosed with lymphedema as well. Pediatric lymphedema is relatively rare, but significantly under-diagnosed and under-treated; it can often be hard for families to find resources and the best possible treatment options for their child. As with adult cases, pediatric lymphedema carries with it the lifelong commitment of having to manage the chronic swelling and prevent secondary complications. Children with lymphedema may be affected by swelling of an extremity (88-96%, most common in the legs), the genitalia (6-14%; most common in combination with leg lymphedema), or other tissue areas.

As with adults, pediatric lymphedema can be classified as primary or secondary pediatric lymphedema, with the primary variant being most common at 97%, to include Milroy's and Meige's disease (see also 2.3 Primary Lymphedema).

The majority of pediatric cases develops symptoms in the infant stage (age 0-1; 49.2%) and during adolescence (age 9-21; 41.3%); early childhood lymphedema (age 1-9; 9.5%) is less prevalent. Boys generally develop symptoms in infancy, whereas most girls present with lymphedema during adolescence[11, 12].

Secondary primary lymphedema can be acquired by surgery involving the lymphatic system, cancer therapy with secondary trauma to the lymphatic system, burn injuries, and other injury.

The treatment of pediatric lymphedema is fundamentally the same as that for the adult patient; however, big emphasis is placed on the education, involvement and communication with the parents and/or caregivers of the child. Parents and caregivers are the best advocates for their child and need to be intimately involved in the treatment and monitoring of the symptoms associated with lymphedema, to include teaching and encouragement of self-management techniques and physical activities.

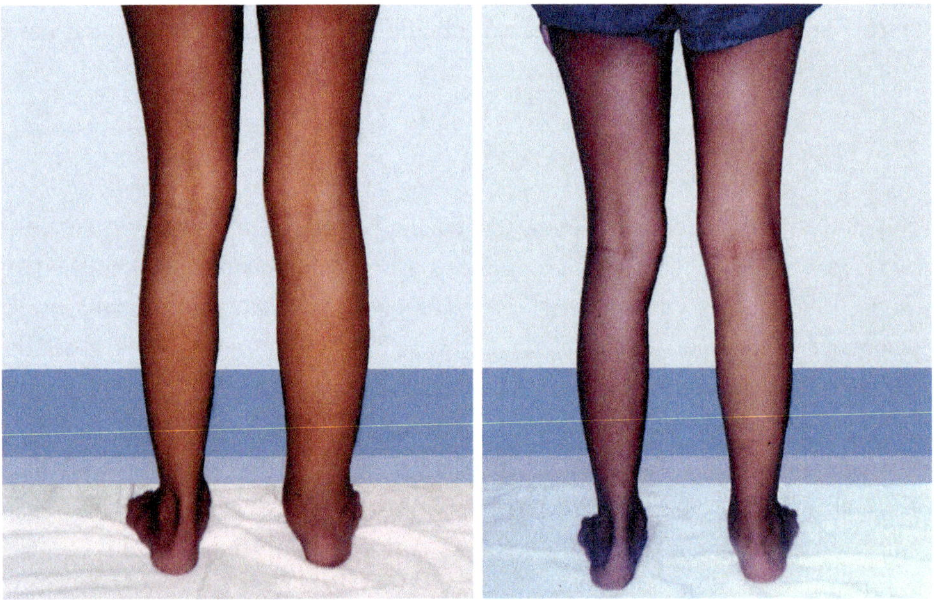

Fig 2.4 Primary adolescent lymphedema of the right leg before (L) and after (R) treatment with Complete Decongestive Therapy. From Zuther J, Norton S Lymphedema Management, 4th ed. Thieme Publishers Stuttgart /New York (reprinted with permission)

Pediatric lymphedema is treated with Complete Decongestive Therapy (CDT; see Treatment section), which needs to be modified accordingly, especially the compression and exercise components of CDT. As with adult cases, pediatric lymphedema will progress if left untreated, and early treatment intervention is imperative in order to avoid further complications.

Pediatric patients should be treated by lymphedema therapists with experience in the treatment of the pediatric population. Resources for parents are sparse, however, one resource offering support and free information is Brylan's Feat Foundation based in Arizona. In addition to providing valuable assistance to parents and caregivers, this foundation offers annual treatment camps for pediatric patients.

2.5 Stages of Lymphedema

Regardless of its classification as primary or secondary, chronic lymphedema is considered to be a progressive condition and cannot simply be described as an accumulation of protein-rich fluid in the tissues of the body. It is a chronic degenerative and inflammatory process affecting the soft tissues, skin, lymph vessels and nodes and may result in severe and often disabling swelling. If lymphedema is left untreated, it progresses through stages over time increasing in size and developing secondary complications[3]. Treatment intervention in early stages (stage 0 and stage I) has been shown to result in very good treatment outcomes if managed appropriately[13].

There are four stages of lymphedema:

2.5.1 Stage 0; Latent or Sub-Clinical Stage

In this stage the extremity appears clinically normal, but the transport capacity of the lymphatic system is reduced; however, the remaining lymph vessels are sufficient to manage the flow of lymph, and swelling is not (yet) visibly present.

Examples include individuals who underwent surgeries for malignancies, such as breast cancer, cancer affecting the genitourinary and gynecologic systems, cancers in the head and neck region, melanoma, or soft tissue malignancies. These procedures generally include the removal of lymph nodes with subsequent disruption of lymphatic pathways.

A condition known as *lymphangiopathy* is present if the reduction in the transport capacity of the lymphatic system is caused by pathology affecting the lymphatic system directly in form of a developmental abnormality (malformations, as in primary lymphedema). In this case lymphedema is not clinically present if the lymphatic system is able to cope.

In this early stage patients may experience early symptoms, such as the feeling of numbness, tingling or fullness in a limb, which is often accompanied by low-grade discomfort. It may be difficult to fit into clothing, and watches, rings or bracelets may feel tight. This sub-clinical stage can exist for months, or years, before any more serious signs appear. The onset of lymphedema correlates to the ability of the lymphatic system to compensate for the reduced transport capacity and any added stress to the system that may cause an increase in the volume of lymphatic fluid.

Treatment intervention in this early and easily manageable stage has been shown to result in very good treatment outcomes using simple, non-custom compression garments[(14)].

2.5.2 Stage 1

Body parts such as the arms or legs are visibly swollen as protein-rich fluid starts to accumulate in the tissues during this stage, which is also known as the pitting, or reversible stage. In many cases, the swelling recedes with elevation, and the extremity may appear normal in the morning; however, as soon as the limb is in a dependent position, the swelling returns. Pitting is easily induced by pressing with the thumb, and the indentation produced by this pressure is retained for some time.

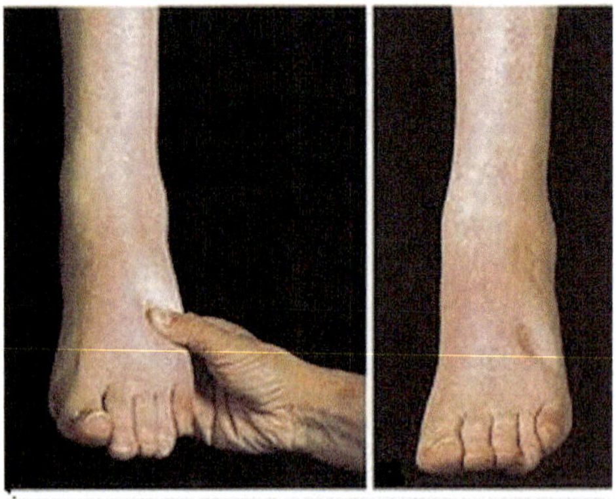

Fig. 2.5 Pitting

Pitting is generally tested on the lower end of the extremity, preferably over bony prominences, and occurs as a result to the displacement of fluid in the tissue caused by pressure applied with the flat thumb. In this stage, fibrotic changes in the tissue are minimal, which is the reason why the indentation produced by the pressure may remain visible over some time. While an increase in fibrous and adipose tissue may be present, this early stage of lymphedema is considered reversible because the skin and tissues have not yet been permanently damaged. Since the swelling appears both marginal and intermittent, patients and medical professionals often deny the need for clinical intervention in this stage; however, with early and appropriate management it is possible to expect reduction of the extremity to a normal size, compared with the uninvolved limb, and to protect the affected body part from progression. Without proper treatment, progression to the next stage is unavoidable in most of the cases.

2.5.3 Stage 2

It is important to point out that the stage of lymphedema is not defined by size, but rather by the consistency of the tissues.

This stage is primarily identified by new formation of fibrotic tissue and additional deposits of fat (fibro-adipose proliferation) with subsequent thickening and hardening of the soft tissues in the skin and subcutis.

In many cases the swelling increases, and elevation of the limb rarely reduces the swelling; pitting is evident (Fig. 2.5). Over time, the tissue continues to harden, and in most cases the Stemmer sign, which is a physical examination finding, becomes positive. A positive Stemmer sign is indicative for lymphedema beginning in the second stage and is tested by pinching and lifting the skin on the back of the fingers or toes[16].

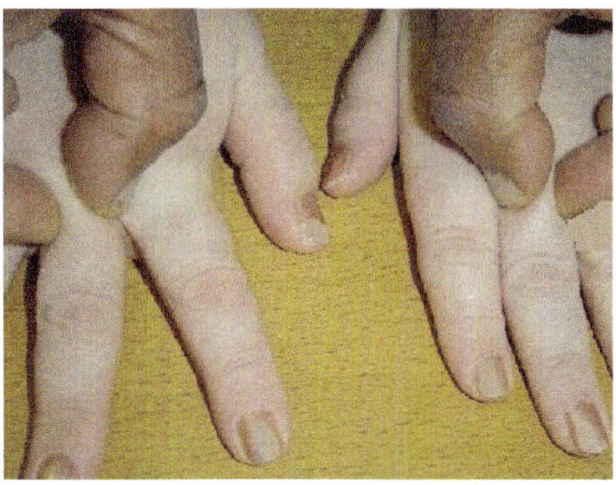

Fig. 2.6 Positive Stemmer sign right hand

In lymphedema, the skin fold produced is thicker and can't be lifted, or lifted only with difficulties compared with the side not affected by lymphedema (Fig. 2.6), which is caused by deposits of fibrotic tissue.

A reduction in volume can be expected if proper treatment is initiated in this stage. In most cases, the excess fibrotic tissue typical in this stage will not recede during the intensive phase of therapy. Reduction in tissue fibrosis is mainly achieved in the second phase of treatment with Complete Decongestive Therapy with proper compression and good patient compliance.

2.5.4 Stage 3

Lymphedema often stabilizes in stage 2. However, if lymphedema remains untreated, protein-rich fluid continues to accumulate, leading to further increase of the swelling, in some cases resulting in extreme proportions. In stage 3 of lymphedema, which is also known as *lymphostatic elephantiasis*, hardening of the tissue continues, evident by a more pronounced Stemmer sign, and further deposition of fat is present. In this stage, pitting is often absent and other changes in the skin, such as benign epithelial growths (papillomas), cysts containing lymphatic fluid, and infections of the nails and the skin develop frequently.

Secondary to the chronic swelling, the body part becomes a perfect culture medium for bacteria and subsequent recurrent infections (lymphangitis) are a common complication. Moreover, untreated lymphedema can lead into a decrease, or loss of functioning of the affected extremity, skin breakdown and sometimes irreversible complications.

Reduction can still be expected if treatment starts in this stage. In most cases the duration of the intensive phase of Complete Decongestive Therapy, as well as any additional treatment modalities, has to be extended and repeated several times. In extreme cases the surgical removal of excess skin following the conservative therapy may be indicated[(17)].

2.6 Complications in Lymphedema

2.6.1 Infections

There are numerous reasons why patients with lymphedema are at an increased risk for infections.

Normally the body is protected by a fine acid layer on the surface of the skin, which prevents bacteria and other pathogens from entering. However, the skin in lymphedema tends to be dry and scaly, causing a disruption of the protective acid layer; if deepened skin folds are present, moisture collecting in these folds may create a breeding ground for bacteria.

The fact that the swelling present in lymphedema causes a disruption of the local immune defense in the affected tissues further complicates this situation. Once bacteria are able to enter the tissue affected by lymphedema, protein and accumulated waste products present in lymphedema provide an ideal breeding ground for infection. Due to the swelling, even in minimal lymphedema, the body's natural defense cells may not be able to fight these invaders sufficiently.

Other complicating factors in lymphedema that can cause infections include lymphatic cysts and lymphorrhea (see 2.6.2).

The initial onset of lymphedema, as well as the worsening of present lymphedema, is frequently associated with the occurrence of infections. It is thought that these infections result in increased fibrosis of lymph vessels and lymph nodes, thus further complicating lymphedema.

Common infections include:

Cellulitis

This is an acute infection of the deeper layers of the skin, which is characterized by painful swelling, redness of the skin, and heat.

Cellulitis is frequently caused by streptococcus and staphylococcus bacteria, which enter the tissues through the skin via cuts, abrasions or breaks. These bacteria are present in the normal skin flora and do not cause an infection while on the healthy skins outer surface.

Cellulitis may become life threatening when it spreads via the lymphatic or blood system to vital organs and other body parts.

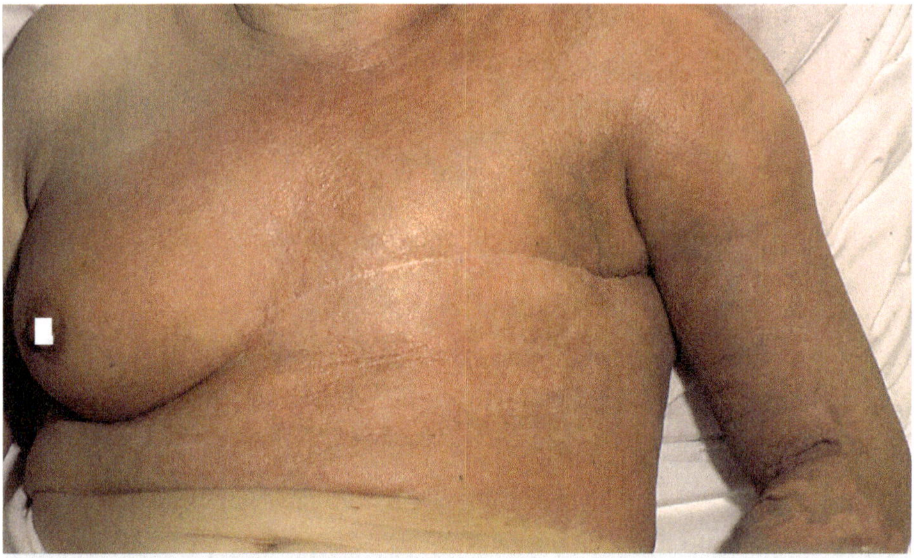

Fig. 2.7 Cellulitis affecting the left arm and thorax of a patient with lymphedema of the left arm. From Zuther J, Norton S Lymphedema Management, 4th ed. Thieme Publishers Stuttgart /New York (reprinted with permission)

Erysipelas

This acute dermal infection is also caused by streptococcus bacteria and affects the skin (more superficial than cellulitis) and tissues located just underneath the skin, to include lymphatic vessels and nodes.

Erysipelas is one of the most common infections in lymphedema and tends to recur. Typical for this infection is its rapid onset, accompanied by fiery red edema with raised and distinct margins in the affected area, and its rapid spreading through superficial lymph vessels, which contributes to the formation of fibrosis in the affected tissues.

Typical symptoms include swelling, redness, fever, headache, sometimes vomiting and chills.

Lymphangitis

Lymphangitis is an infection of the lymphatic vessels and most often results from an acute streptococcal infection of the skin, which is regularly associated with cellulitis. Less frequently it results from a staphylococcal infection.

The infection may spread to the blood stream causing a potentially life-threatening emergency. Symptoms include visible red streaks from the infected area to the armpit or groin, fever, pain, headache and enlarged lymph nodes.

Individuals who are at a high risk for lymphedema must remain alert to the signs of infection as these symptoms are often indicative for the onset of lymphedema. In such cases, quick intervention may help to delay the onset of lymphedema, as well as prevent the infection. The problem may aggravate and become potentially life threatening if timely care is not taken.

In case of infections, antibiotics should be administered as soon as possible; penicillin-based medications are used either orally, if no systemic infection is present, or by intravenous application. Other antibiotics may be used in cases of penicillin allergy. In severe cases hospitalization may be necessary. In some patients, prophylactic antibiotic therapy may be used to prevent recurrent infections in patients with lymphedema[18].

Lymphedema patients with a history of recurrent infections should have a two-week supply of antibiotics on hand, particularly while traveling.

Treatment should be suspended during episodes of acute infection and fever. In order to prevent excessive swelling, light compression should be applied during these episodes if tolerated.

2.6.2 Leaking of Lymph Fluid

The leakage or weeping of high-protein lymph fluid from the tissues onto the surface of the skin, which usually manifests as a beading or trickling of fluid, is also known as *lymphorrhea*. It is more common in the legs and genital areas, especially if prolonged restriction in mobility is an issue, but can also affect other areas of the body, for example in the axillary area.

The leaking fluid is usually clear and colorless (sometimes straw or amber-colored, or milky) if it appears in isolation. If lymphorrhea appears in the presence of wound secretion (exudate), its color and consistency will be dictated by the exudate.

Lymphorrhea often appears as a complication following the removal of axillary or inguinal lymph nodes; it can also be present in lymphedema following minor trauma to the swollen area, especially in vulnerable skin of the elderly or in palliative patients.

Any trauma to the skin, which may be caused by insect bites, cuts, abrasions, cracks in dry skin, has the potential to allow lymph to weep onto the skin surface. In some cases, lymphorrhea may be the result of a ruptured lymph cysts (lymphocele), which is an abnormal blister-like collection of lymphatic fluid on the skin as a result of injured lymph vessels, often following surgical procedures (Fig. 2.8).

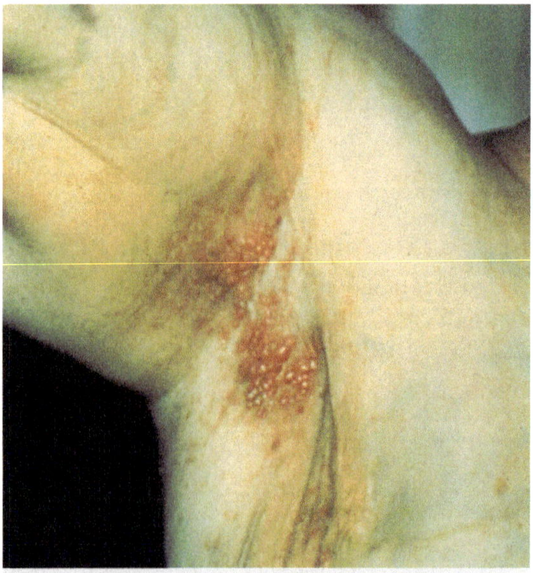

Fig. 2.8 Lymphatic cysts in the right axilla. From Zuther J, Norton S Lymphedema Management, 4th ed. Thieme Publishers Stuttgart /New York (reprinted with permission)

While the leakage is often associated with known causes, as described above, it may also start spontaneously, seemingly out of nowhere, most likely due to high pressure of lymph fluid inside the skin tissues. The skin is often so tense with excess fluid that it is unable to stretch fast enough to accommodate the fluid, causing it to split or tear with the slightest bump or nick, resulting in lymphorrhea. The discharge may be mild or excessive, leading to wetness in clothing, compression garments or bandages, footwear, and bedding.

The presence of lymphorrhea can cause secondary complications, such as infections (cellulitis), and further breakdown of the skin, caused by excessive moisture. If lymphorrhea is present in combination with chronic wounds, the caustic nature of the exudating fluid associated with lymphorrhea is known to be destructive to the wound bed, which can lead to more increased and widespread ulceration.

In order to stop the leakage and to prevent further complications, it is important to initiate treatment immediately. Trained health care professionals and certified lymphedema therapists involved in the care of lymphedema, should be able to initiate proper treatment following a full assessment of the cause for the leakage.

In order to stop the fluid from leaking and to promote healing of the skin damage, a series of steps are essential:

The area where the fluid is leaking needs to be cleaned carefully and thoroughly with soap and water to reduce risk of infection. Following this, a moisturizing cream or lotion should be applied to the skin to improve the condition and protect it from further breakdown. The leaking area should then be covered with a sterile, non-adherent and absorbent dressing to prevent further trauma to the skin and to absorb he leaking fluid.

The main component to stop lymphorrhea is compression, which is administered by padded short-stretch compression bandages, which are applied on top of the dressing and may have to be replaced frequently during the first 2-3 days to remove wet bandages and dressings. It is important to point out that the entire swollen area (for example the entire leg) must be covered with bandages in order to prevent a tourniquet-like effect and subsequent accumulation of fluid below the area affected by lymphorrhea. In addition, the extremity should be elevated as much as possible to reduce the effects of gravity and assist venous and lymphatic drainage.

Following these steps will improve the skin condition and stop the leakage within 2-3 days in most cases, at which point the regular compression garment should again be applied.

2.6.3 Axillary Web Syndrome

A number of patients who underwent axillary lymph node dissection (ALND) in combination with breast cancer or melanoma surgery experience postoperative pain and limited range of motion associated with a palpable cord of tissue extending from the axilla into the arm on the same side. This condition is known as Axillary Web Syndrome (AWS)[19,20], which usually occurs within 2 and 8 weeks following surgery; however, it has also been identified in patients months to years after surgery[20,21]. The incidence of AWS ranges from 6-72%[20].

AWS appears as a cord of tissue just underneath the skin located in the axilla and may run down the inside of the arm towards the elbow. It occasionally extends down as far as the hand near the thumb and has also been identified along the side of the trunk underneath the arm. Restrictions in movement and pain often accompany this condition.

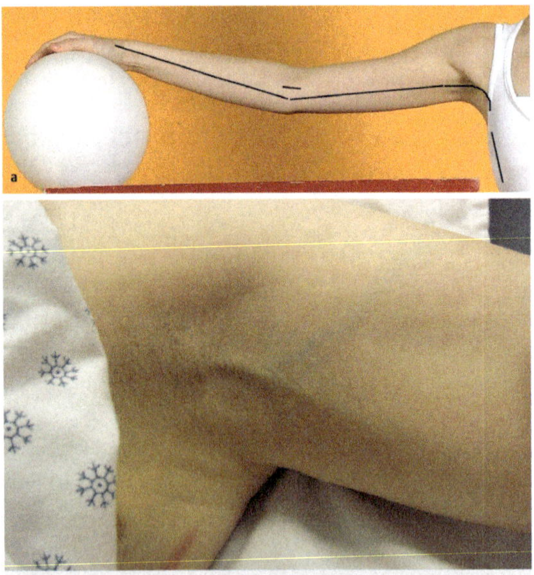

Fig. 2.9 (a) Location of AWS. (b) AWS left axilla. From Zuther J, Norton S Lymphedema Management, 4th ed. Thieme Publishers Stuttgart /New York (reprinted with permission)

The cord becomes tight with movement of the arm especially with shoulder abduction (bringing the arm out to the side). If the cord runs down the arm, elbow extension (straightening the elbow) and wrist movements can also be limited in addition to restricted movements of the trunk.

A person with AWS tends to experience pain and pulling sensation with movement of the arm, especially shoulder abduction because this movement puts tension on the cord. There is usually little to no pain when the arm is at rest. It is common for a person to have good movement in the arm following surgery, however, movement becomes limited and painful when the AWS cord begins to develop. The sudden onset of pain and limited movement may lead to anxiety and stress in someone who is already dealing with a cancer diagnosis. AWS appears to occur more often in people who are slimmer for reasons unknown(19,20). The cord is often easier to identify in a person with a slim build since there is less fatty tissue to conceal the cord. It is possible AWS is present in heavier patients, but the cord is not detectable because it is covered by fatty tissue.

The cause of AWS is still unknown but appears to be associated with lymph node removal therefore having a possible lymphatic involvement.

The literature reports a higher incidence of AWS and a more extensive AWS cord with a higher number of lymph nodes removed(19,20). The AWS cord also appears to extend further down the arm in patients with more lymph nodes removed. It is speculated the cord is caused by a blockage in a vessel, lymphatic or venous, or by tightness in the surrounding tissue(19,21). Biopsies of the cord have identified it as being a vessel, both lymphatic and venous, with more evidence suggesting lymphatic vessel involvement(19,21). More research is needed to identify the underlying cause and physiology of AWS.

Some people are of the opinion that AWS completely resolves on its own within about three months after surgery, therefore treatment is not necessary(19). Others believe the cord may not completely go away, which may lead to long term movement restrictions and functional problems(23,24).

Pain medications such as non-steroidal anti-inflammatory drugs (NSAIDS) may be recommended dependent on the amount of associated pain(25). Since pain is often experienced with certain movements, some patients will avoid moving the arm. Lack of movement could lead to secondary problems such as soft tissue tightness and joint problems; therefore avoiding movement is not recommended. Movement of the arm is encouraged but minimal to no pain should be experienced during the movement.

Rehabilitation treatment such as physical therapy has been used to treat the movement restrictions caused by the cord(20,23,26-29). The techniques include gentle stretching of the cord and surrounding muscles and soft tissue to improve movement. Manual techniques have been described as skin traction, cord bending, myofascial release, soft tissue mobilization, and scar releases.

Gentle manual techniques are recommended to avoid lymphedema or reddening of the skin. At times, the cord has been reported to break with manual techniques which results in an immediate increase in movement. The breaking of the cord may be felt and heard by the patient and/or therapist. It is not known what exactly is breaking, but it is speculated it could be the cord or the supporting tissue around the cord. It doesn't appear there are any negative effects from breaking the cord since the patient sustains the sudden gain in movement.

It is highly recommended therapists should be cautious when using manual techniques and avoid being too aggressive. Breaking of the cord is mentioned only to inform patients and medical professionals about the possibility of the cord breaking with gentle manual techniques. It is not recommended aggressive treatment techniques be used to purposely break the cord.

Further research is needed to fully understand the phenomenon of AWS, the physiology, and treatment.

2.7 Contributing Pathologies to Lymphedema

2.7.1 Obesity

Successful long-term management of lymphedema also includes the elimination of risk factors that are known to have detrimental effects on lymphedema. One of these risk factors is obesity, which often worsens the symptoms of existing lymphedema. Studies show a significant connection between obesity and the development of upper extremity lymphedema following breast cancer surgery[30-32] and the correlation between body mass index (BMI) and change in the development of lymphedema[33].

Excessive weight and obesity may also contribute to the onset of primary and secondary lymphedema involving the lower extremities. Excessive weight, especially morbid obesity can have a negative impact on the return of lymphatic fluid from the legs; additional fluid volumes associated with obesity may overwhelm an already impaired lymphatic system. Direct pressure on lymphatic vessels by excess fatty tissue, impaired diaphragmatic breathing and decreased muscular function can also be factors contributing to the manifestation of lymphedema.

Chronic venous insufficiency (CVI; see 2.7.2) is often associated with obesity. The increased burden on the lymphatic system in CVI can play a significant role in the manifestation of lower extremity lymphedema.

Treatment progress in existing lymphedema may be hampered in patients with a high BMI. With obese patients it is often difficult to apply bandages, especially in cases of lymphedema affecting the lower extremities. Furthermore, the compressive materials (bandages, garments) applied to the affected extremities tend to slide in cases of obesity. Compression garments may have to be custom ordered, creating an additional financial burden to the patient.

Exercise is an important aspect in the successful management of lymphedema and may be negatively affected by a high BMI as well. Mobility problems associated with a high body mass index can affect the patients' participation in treatment, and exercise protocols used in lymphedema therapy for the upper and lower extremities may have to be modified accordingly.

Weight management and proper nutrition are essential for successful long-term lymphedema management.

2.7.2 Chronic Venous Insufficiency

Chronic venous insufficiency (CVI) is an advanced stage of venous disease that occurs when the inner lining of the veins and/or the valves located within the larger veins are not working sufficiently, causing venous blood to collect or "pool" in the veins, which is known as venous stasis. If treatment of CVI is neglected, lymphedema may develop as a result in the later stages of this condition. Late stage CVI (phlebo-lymphedema) is considered to be the most common cause for lymphedema in the Western world[34].

The blood pressure inside the thin-walled veins is considerably lower than the pressure in the arteries. In healthy veins, a system of valves inside the larger veins prevents pooling of venous blood in the lower extremities and helps to ensure the efficient transport the venous blood back to the heart. A sufficient return of venous blood to the heart would not be possible without the help of the muscle and joint pumps, diaphragmatic breathing and the suction effect of the heart during its relaxation phase (diastole). Together with a functioning valvular system in the veins, these supporting mechanisms propel the venous blood back to the heart.

Chronic venous insufficiency develops most commonly as a result of blood clots in the deeper veins of the legs. This condition, known as deep venous thrombosis (DVT), results in changes in the fluid dynamics in the veins and causes the pressure in the veins to increase, and the system of valves to become insufficient. If the venous blood pressure stays elevated over long periods of time, chronic venous insufficiency develops. Chronic venous insufficiency resulting from DVT is also known as post-thrombotic syndrome; as many as 14% of individuals affected by DVT will develop this problem within five years after diagnosis[35].

The problems associated with CVI do not disappear without treatment and the complexity of treatment increases as the disease progresses. Untreated CVI can lead to complications, to include lymphedema, and early diagnosis and treatment is of utmost importance. A specialized physician should be consulted as soon as the following symptoms are present:

- Swelling in the lower legs and ankles, especially after extended periods of standing. This is often the first sign and caused by the pooling of venous blood
- Heavy, tired, aching or restless legs
- New varicose veins
- Leathery-looking skin on the legs
- Flaking or itching skin on the legs or feet
- Stasis ulcers (or venous stasis ulcers) generally around the ankles, that won't heal

These symptoms are caused by a condition known as ambulatory venous hypertension, which is a result of obstruction inside veins, retrograde (backward) venous flow (venous reflux), or a combination of these.

The deficient valves in the veins in CVI fail to prevent the retrograde flow of venous blood during muscle pump activity, specifically the activity of the calf musculature during walking (ambulatory). Muscle activity in the legs applies outside pressure to the veins and a functioning system of valves forces the venous blood upward and towards the heart while walking and prevents back flow. In CVI the blood is not only forced upward towards the heart during muscle activity, but also "backwards" causing the pressure in the veins of the lower leg to increase even more (ambulatory venous hypertension).

This pathological increase in pressure subsequently affects the blood capillaries, and more fluid is filtered from the blood into the tissues. The lymphatic system is responsible for the compensation of the increased amount of tissue fluid and will increase its activity; this is also known as the lymphatic safety function. If the lymphatic system, despite working to its maximum capacity, is not able to cope with the additional fluid, swelling (edema) develops in the leg.

In the initial stages this swelling may recede with elevation and rest, but over time and without adequate treatment (compression, elevation, exercise), the constant strain on the lymphatic system may lead to damage to the lymphatic vessels, leading to reduction of its transport capacity.

This condition, described as combined venous and lymphatic insufficiency, has serious consequences, and without treatment the symptoms associated with CVI and ambulatory venous hypertension will gradually worsen, and the condition will progress through the following stages:

Stage 0

As long as the lymphatic system is able to compensate for the increase in tissue fluid resulting from venous hypertension, affected individuals remain free of edema, but may experience other symptoms typically associated with CVI (see above); this stage is also known as the sub-clinical stage.

Stage 1

The lymphatic system is not yet clinically affected and works to its maximum capacity, but is unable to drain the elevated fluid resulting from the ambulatory venous hypertension. The lymphatic system experiences overload of lymph fluid, which is also known as dynamic insufficiency of the lymphatic system (see 2.2 Insufficiencies of the Lymphatic System).

Edema develops over the course of the day. In the early stages the lymphatic system is able to catch up with the excess fluid in the tissues during rest at night, and the edema tends to decrease or completely recede during nighttime rest. At night the gravitational forces are inactive and the pressure in the venous system returns to normal values in the supine position.

Proper treatment approaches in this stage include elevation, exercises and compression.

Stage 2

Blood capillaries with elevated pressure values, and lymph vessels working on their maximum capacity that remain without appropriate intervention and treatment for extended periods of time, will eventually suffer damage. Red blood cells (erythrocytes) leave the blood capillaries through their stretched walls, causing the skin to become reddish-brown due to deposits of tissue storage iron (hemosiderin).

Subsequent to high pressure inside the lymphatics, the walls of lymph vessels develop fibrosis and the valves inside larger vessels become inefficient, which causes impairment of the lymphatic system to a point so severe that it is unable to perform its basic functions (mechanical insufficiency). This results in an accumulation of not only fluid, but also protein in the tissues.

This stage is described as phlebo-lymphedema; lymphedema will develop as a result of the venous pathology, and its severity is exacerbated by the symptoms associated with CVI. The lymphedema appears initially smooth and is pitting. Without treatment it progresses into a more fibrotic stage (see 2.5, stages of lymphedema). Early diagnosis and treatment are of utmost importance to prevent further complications. Complete Decongestive Therapy is indicated treatment approach in this stage.

Stage 3

Severe changes in the skin and subcutaneous tissues are typical in this stage. Ulcerations may develop secondary to reduced oxygenation and nutrition of the tissues. In addition to lymphedema and leg ulcers, symptoms of lipo-dermatosclerosis are present, which include:

- Pain
- Hardening of the skin
- Localized thickening
- Moderate redness
- Increased pigmentation
- Small white scarred areas
- Varicose veins

In addition to Complete Decongestive Therapy, other treatment approaches, such as wound care, may become necessary.

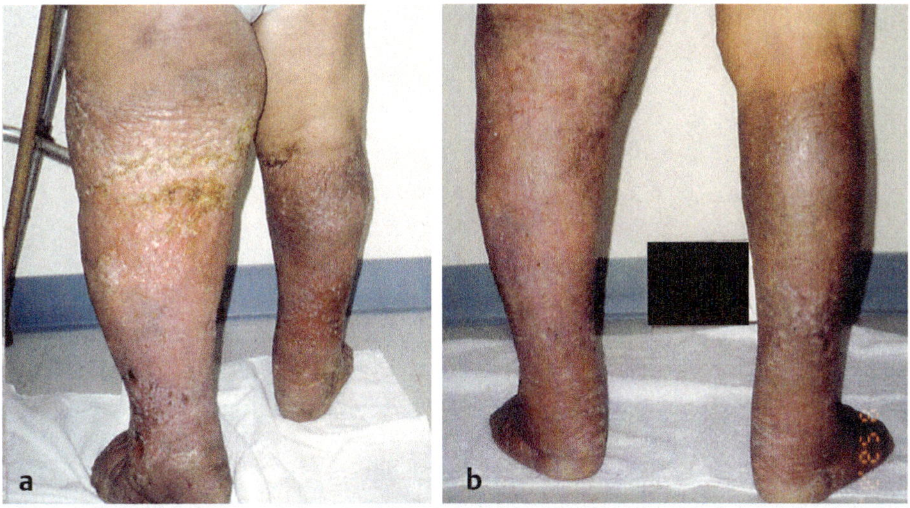

Fig. 2.10 Lymphedema combined with Chronic Venous Insufficiency (stage 3), ulcerations and lymphatic leakage on both legs. (a) before and (b) after Complete Decongestive Therapy. From Zuther J, Norton S Lymphedema Management, 4th ed. Thieme Publishers Stuttgart /New York (reprinted with permission)

2.7.3 Lipedema

Lipedema (fluid in fat) is characterized by symmetric enlargement of the limbs, generally affecting the lower extremities and extending from the hips and buttocks to the ankles secondary to the deposition of fat; upper extremities are affected in 30%[36] of the cases.

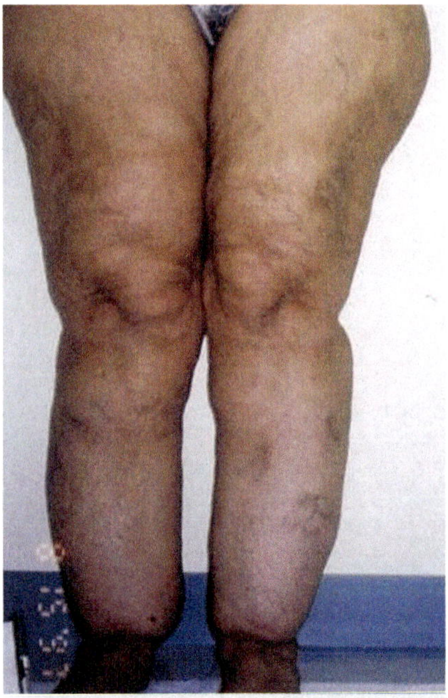

Figure 2.11 Lipedema

Lipedema is not rare and not caused by obesity, or a disorder of the lymphatic system, and is commonly misdiagnosed as bilateral lymphedema, extreme cellulitis, or morbid obesity. Lipedema is a symmetric painful fat disorder.

If lipedema left untreated, it can cause multiple secondary health problems, including mobility and joint issues, non-lipedema obesity, venous insufficiency and lymphedema (lipo-lymphedema). The quality of life in individuals affected by lipedema is often decreased due to the fact that the condition is typically dismissed as simple obesity by clinicians unfamiliar with the symptoms.

Most used synonyms for lipedema include:

Adiposalgia/Adipoalgesia, Adiposis dolorosa, Lipalgia, Lipomatosis dolorosa of the legs, Lipodystrophia dolorosa, or painful column leg.

Lipedema almost exclusively affects women; males are rarely affected[39]. The underlying cause for the development of lipedema remains unknown; it is thought to be associated with hormonal disorders and can be hereditary with 15% of affected individuals having a family history of lipedema[38,40].

Lipedema can develop early in puberty; however, the mean age of diagnosis is around the age of 35.

Lipedema can be diagnosed based on clinical criteria, such as history and typical clinical features, and by physical examination rather than with diagnostic tests.

Clinical Features:

- Symmetrical distribution of fat between the hips and ankles, the feet are not involved
- Ring of fatty tissue overlapping the tops of the feet
- Tissue has a soft rubber-like feel in early stages
- Initially, the skin color is normal
- Typical bulges of fatty tissue on the inner thigh (above the knee and close to the groin) are seen in later stages
- Small fatty lumps (nodules) within the tissues start to form in later stages
- In the early stages of lipedema the upper part of the body is often slender
- Weight loss does not influence the areas affected by lipedema
- Swelling (edema) is common in the second half of the day and includes the feet, but decreases in the early stage with elevation and night-time rest
- Pain, tenderness, sensitivity to pressure
- Easy bruising

Lipedema affects the lymphatic system; the excessive amount of fatty tissue present in lipedema compresses the lymph collectors of the superficial lymphatic system, which are embedded in the fatty subcutaneous tissue. Lymphangiographic imaging shows that the lymph collectors within the increased fatty tissue have a coiled or corkscrew-like appearance rather than passing fairly straight towards the lymph nodes as is the case in healthy tissue. This can result in a reduced transport capacity of the lymphatic system in the affected area.

If the capacity of the lymphatic system is reduced to such an extent that it becomes unable to perform one of its basic functions, the removal of water from the tissues, fluid will accumulate and "real" edema develops in addition to lipedema. In the initial stages, the swelling may recede with elevation and rest, but over time and without adequate treatment (compression, elevation, exercise), the constant strain on the lymphatic system may cause damage to the lymphatic vessels, leading to further reduction of its transport capacity, and constant swelling may be present.

Lipo-lymphedema: As a result of damage to the lymphatic system, lymphedema may develop secondary to lipedema, and is then known as lipo-lymphedema, which increases the complexity of treatment.

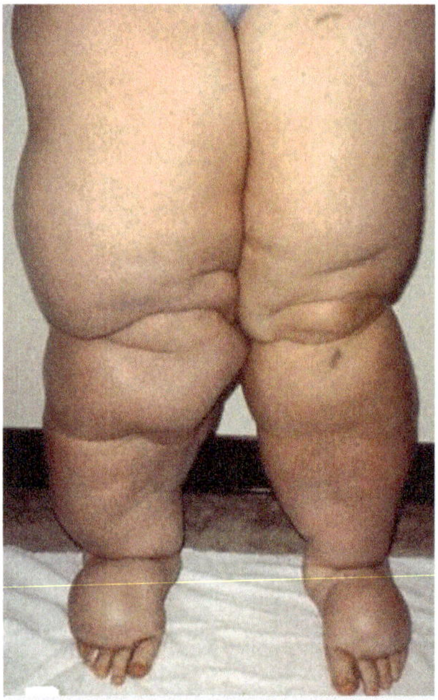

Fig. 2.12 Lipo-lymphedema

If lipo-lymphedema remains without treatment, it will progress through the same stages as primary or secondary lymphedema.

Early diagnosis and treatment for lipedema is important and can determine the individual's long-term prognosis. Therapy for lipedema can be largely divided into conservative treatments to reduce edema, and surgical treatments such as liposuction.

Main goals in the conservative treatment of lipedema are to decrease pain and hypersensitivity, increase mobility and to prevent, or if already present, to address the edema associated with lipedema.

If lipedema, or lipo-lymphedema is associated with obesity, nutritional guidance must be provided to reduce weight and avoid further weight gain [41].

Conservative approaches include Complete Decongestive Therapy (CDT); CDT does not address proliferated fatty tissue but contributes to the reduction of edema and the prevention of the manifestation of lipo-lymphedema.

In most cases, it is necessary to apply a lower level of compression with bandages or compression garments due to pain and hypersensitivity in the affected areas. Compression garments generally have to be custom-made to the individual's measurements. If the use of compression garments is discontinued, edema will return in most cases.

Intermittent pneumatic compression, also known as compression pumps, may also be applied to reduce symptoms associated with lipedema (see 3.3).

Surgical treatment may be considered for patients who do not respond to conservative treatment. Liposuction is currently the standard surgical treatment method; however, this procedure may cause bleeding and secondary damage to lymph vessels resulting in persistent swelling. New and more advanced techniques may reduce these risks; however, individuals considering this approach should ensure that the performing physician is experienced and follows internationally established guidelines.

There is generally an increased tendency for swelling following the surgical procedure, thus CDT should be initiated or continued within a few days of the procedure.

In the presence of additional lymphedema (lipo-lymphedema) the treatment protocol for CDT corresponds with that for primary lymphedema, and shows good long-term results. However, individuals affected by this condition need to understand that, although the lymphatic component responds well to CDT, the reduction of fatty tissue responds more slowly, and sometimes not at all.

Several marked differences between lipedema and lymphedema can be distinguished; these differences are highlighted in the table below.

Table 1 Differences between lipedema and lymphedema

Lipedema	**Lymphedema**
Symmetric (buttocks involved)	Not symmetric
Foot not involved	Foot involved
Not pitting	Pitting edema
Stemmer sign negative	Stemmer sign positive
Tissue feels rubbery	Tissue feels firmer (starting in stage 2 lymphedema)
Painful to touch	Generally not painful to touch
Easy bruising	Generally not bruising
Hormonal disturbances frequent	Generally no hormonal disturbance

2.8 Diagnosis of Lymphedema

An early and correct diagnosis of lymphedema is critical since lymphedema can be treated more effectively the earlier it is diagnosed.

A physician with knowledge of lymphedema is able to establish the diagnosis of lymphedema clinically by taking the patients medical history and performing a physical examination.

The diagnosis of lymphedema includes measuring the circumference of the affected arms or legs to determine the volume of fluid buildup in the affected limbs. Measurements are taken either circumferentially with measuring tape in certain intervals, perometry (a computer based infrared optical electronic scanner), or volume displacement (the extremity is placed in a container filled with water, and the amount of the displaced water determines the volume of lymphedema when compared to the unaffected extremity; accurate but rarely used).

The physician determines whether symptoms, such as swelling in the arms or legs, might be caused by other conditions, including blood clots, or cardiac insufficiencies, which are treated differently. To further establish the diagnosis, certain imaging tests may be performed in order to conclude the exact cause of the fluid buildup in the tissues.

These tests may include:

Lymphoscintigraphy

This highly sensitive imaging method is specific for lymphedema. It is most commonly performed in the diagnosis of this condition and considered to be highly accurate in the detection of lymphatic dysfunction associated with lymphedema[(42).]

Lymphoscintigraphy involves the injection of a radioactive tracer protein into the skin at the lower end (often the web spaces of fingers and toes) of the affected extremity. The tracer is absorbed by the lymphatic system and travels inside lymph collectors to the regional lymph nodes of the extremity (axillary and inguinal lymph nodes). A specialized camera detects the signal given off by the radiotracer on their way to the lymph nodes, which enables the physician to evaluate the severity of the lymphatic dysfunction in lymphedema.

Bioimpedance Spectroscopy (BIS)

Bioimpedance spectroscopy is an effective tool to detect lymphedema early. Bioimpedance measurements are taken by sending a harmless, painless low-frequency electrical current through the body fluids and measuring the body's resistance (or impedance) to this electrical current. The resistance of the body fluids to the electrical current is inverse proportion to the volume of extracellular fluid, which means that the higher the volume, the lower the resistance. As lymphedema develops, the amount of fluid will increase, making it easier for the signal to travel though the extracellular fluid of the body.

In the clinical setting, the BIS device measures the resistance of the unaffected limb and compares the result to the resistance of the affected (or at risk) limb, which is expressed as the "impedance ratio", or the L-Dex score. The L-Dex score represents the difference in the amount of extracellular fluid present in lymphedema compared to an unaffected limb.

An L-Dex unit change of 6.5 from baseline suggests that sub-clinical lymphedema is present, and an L-Dex unit change of 7.0 or more from baseline is an indication that clinical lymphedema is present[43], and that the patient should be referred to lymphedema therapy.

In general, it can be said that the higher the L-Dex score, the more severe the symptoms of lymphedema.

MRI Scan

By using a strong magnetic field and radio waves, detailed 3-D images of the involved body parts are produced, and lymphatic trunks, collectors and nodes are visualized.

CT Scan

This technique produces detailed cross-sectional images of the affected body parts and can detect blockages in the lymphatic system. It can also detect any possible new tissue formations (tumors) that may obstruct parts of the lymphatic system.

MRI and CT scans are expensive and are generally used to detect malignant tumors.

Ultrasound

Ultrasound is a simple, non-invasive test that can identify lymphedema by specific tissue characteristics. This test uses high frequency sound waves to produce images of internal structures. It can help find obstructions within the lymphatic system and vascular system and is often used to detect abnormal venous conditions, such as deep venous thrombosis, which can be a cause for lymphedema (see 2.7.2).

2.9 Lymphedema and it's Impact on the Quality of Life

The considerable psychological and social impact of chronic lymphedema on the quality of life (QoL) and well-being of patients around the globe affected by this disease is known and confirmed in the literature for quite some time[43-45,53].

The highest incidence of secondary lymphedema in the United States is observed following surgery and radiation for malignancies, particularly among those individuals affected by breast cancer, which is conceivably the reason why most of the research on the impact of lymphedema on QoL was conducted on survivors of breast cancer with subsequent lymphedema. This research indicates that health-related QoL was significantly lower in breast cancer patients with diagnosed lymphedema, or with arm symptoms without diagnosed lymphedema, compared with patients without lymphedema or arm symptoms[46].

Any woman treated for breast cancer has a risk of developing lymphedema during or after the surgical/radiation/chemotherapy treatment necessary to eradicate the tumor.

The impact of these procedures on the sufficiency of the lymphatic system may result in the onset of lymphedema in almost half of the affected women.

However, the literature also shows that the QoL of individuals affected by primary lymphedema and other forms of secondary lymphedema is negatively affected as well by this chronic condition. Several studies indicate that patients affected by chronic edema of the lower extremities reported a higher impact on QoL than individuals with upper extremity lymphedema(47-49).

It is also important to point out that the negative effects on QoL of lymphedema in many cases extends to the families of those living and coping with chronic edema(50, 51).

As soon as, and sometimes before the swelling is present, patients are confronted by aesthetic problems (skin changes, increase in extremity size, ill-fitting clothing), functional problems (pain, stiffness, numbness, functional limitations, limitations in range of motion in the affected extremity, compromised normal activities of daily living and occupational responsibilities), psychological problems (negative self-identity, emotional disturbance, stress, negative impact on family life, social isolation, perceived reduced sexuality), as well as financial impact.

When some patients realize that lymphedema is a chronic disease that requires life-long management, these problems may intensify, and patients feel that coping with the swelling is more demanding than the treatment of the disease that caused lymphedema in the first place.

To effectively combat not only the swelling, but also the negative impact of lymphedema on psycho-social well-being, early diagnosis, evaluation, and coordinated multi-disciplinary treatment strategies by certified lymphedema therapists and qualified health care professionals is imperative.

By definition, the goal of all treatment is to improve the patient's state of health; addressing the QoL consequences of the patient has an important role to play alongside the objective of reducing limb volume.

Studies indicate that QoL improves with a reduction in limb volume(52); early diagnosis and subsequent efficient therapeutic intervention for lymphedema is, therefore, crucial to optimal treatment outcomes. However, effective lymphedema management should not only include comprehensive treatment by qualified health care providers to reduce the swelling, combined with education of the patients regarding self-care measures; it should also address the QoL consequences of the disease and improve health-related QoL and psychological well-being by evaluating psychological and psychosocial criteria and educating the patient on support groups and interactive support.

In addition to treating the lymphedema, the lymphedema therapist plays an important role in educating the patient regarding the treatment measures and self-care techniques (Self-MLD, self-bandaging, skin, and nail care, etc.).

Oftentimes patients have a hard time accepting the need for the application of bulky padded compression bandages on the affected extremity during the intensive phase of Complete Decongestive Therapy (CDT). Compression bandages are necessary to address the fluctuating volume of the lymphedema during this intensive phase, in which the patient is treated ideally daily. To reduce anxiety and improve patient compliance, it is crucial for the patient to know, that the need for compression bandages is only temporary. Once the swollen body part is decongested and the patient transitions into phase two of CDT (self-management phase), the bandages will be replaced by fitted compression garments.

References

(1) Petrek JA, Senie RT, Peters M, et al. Lymphedema in a cohort of breast carcinoma survivors 20 years after diagnosis. Cancer. 2001;92:1368-77.

(2) US Breast Cancer Statistics. Retrieved from www.breastcancer.org/facts-statistics (accessed May 2022)

(3) Arin K. Greene, Jeremy A. Goss Diagnosis and Staging of Lymphedema Semin Plast Surg. 2018 Feb; 32(1): 12–16. Published online 2018 Apr 9. doi: 10.1055/s-0038-1635117 PMCID: PMC5891654

(4) Ferrell R, Kimak M, Lawrence E, Finegold D Candidate gene analysis

in primary lymphedema. Lymphat Res Biol .2008;6(2):69-76.doi: 10.1089/lrb.2007.1022

(5) Schook C, et al. Primary lymphedema: clinical features and management in 138 pediatric patients Plast Reconstr Surg .2011 Jun;127(6):2419-2431. doi:10.1097/PRS.0b013e318213a218.

(6) Brouillard P et al. Non-hotspot PIK3CA mutations are more frequent in CLOVES than in common or combined lymphatic malformations. Orphanet J Rare Dis 2021 Jun 10;16(1):267.doi: 10.1186/s13023-021-01898-y.

(7) Al-Olabi L et al. Mosaic RAS/MAPK variants cause sporadic vascular malformations which respond to targeted therapy. J Clin Invest .2018 Apr 2;128(4):1496-1508.doi: 10.1172/JCI98589.Epub 2018 Mar 12.

(8) Syaza Hazwany A et al. The Unresolved Pathophysiology of Lymphedema. Front. Physiol., 17 March 2020 https://doi.org/10.3389/fphys.2020.00137

(9) Fu M et al. The effect of providing information about lymphedema on the cognitive and symptom outcomes of breast cancer survivors. Ann Surg Oncol.2010 Jul;17(7):1847-53.doi: 10.1245/s10434-010-0941-3.Epub 2010 Feb 6.

(10) Gupta S S, Mayrovitz H N (April 03, 2022) The Breast Edema Enigma: Features, Diagnosis, Treatment, and Recommendations. Cureus 14(4): e23797. doi:10.7759/cureus.23797

(11) Todd J., Craig G., Todd M., et al. Audit of childhood lymphoedema in the United Kingdom undertaken by members of the Children's Lymphoedema Special Interest Group. J of Lymphoedema. 2014;9(2):14-19.

(12) Schook C.C., Mulliken J.B., Fishman S.J. et al. Primary lymphedema: clinical features and management in 138 pediatric patients. Plast Reconstr Surg. 2011 Jun;127(6):2419-31.

(13) Torres Lacompa, M, Yuse Sanches, MJ, et al.(2010) Effectiveness of early physiotherapy to prevent lymphedema after surgery for breast cancer: randomized, single blinded, clinical trial, *BMJ,* 340:b5397.

(14) Stout Gergich NL, Pfalzer LA, McGarvey C, Springer B, Gerber LH, Soballe P. (2008) Preoperative assessment enables the early diagnosis and successful treatment of lymphedema. *Cancer*, 112:2809-2819.

(15) Levenhagen K, Davies C, Perdomo M, Ryans K, Gilchrist L. Diagnosis of Upper Quadrant Lymphedema Secondary to Cancer: Clinical Practice Guideline From the Oncology Section of the American Physical Therapy Association. *Physical Therapy*, Volume 97, Issue 7, July 2017, Pages 729–745, https://doi.org/10.1093/ptj/pzx050

(16) Goss J, Greene A. Sensitivity and Specificity of the Stemmer Sign for Lymphedema: A Clinical Lymphoscintigraphic Study. Plast Reconstr Surg Glob Open._2019 Jun; 7(6)

(17) Kareh A, Kyle Y. Surgical Management of Lymphedema. Journal List Mo Med v.117(2); Mar-Apr 2020 PMC7144713

(18) Should prophylactic antibiotic therapy be used to prevent recurrent infection in patients with lymphedema? HemOnc Today. November 10, 2017 Issue

(19) Moskovitz AH, Anderson BO, Yeung RS, Byrd DR, Lawton TJ, Moe RE. Axillary web syndrome after axillary dissection.*Am J Surg*. 2001;181(5):434-439.

(20) Koehler LA et al. Axillary web syndrome following breast cancer surgery: symptoms, complications, and management strategies. Breast Cancer (Dove Med Press).2019; 11: 13–19.Published online 2018 Dec 20.doi:10.2147/ BCTT.S146635

(21) O'Toole J et al. Cording Following Treatment for Breast Cancer. Breast Cancer Res Treat. 2013 Jul; 140(1): 105–111. Published online 2013 Jun 29.doi:10.1007/s10549-013-2616-9

(22) Reedijk M, Boerner S, Ghazarian D, McCready D. A case of axillary web syndrome with subcutaneous nodules following axillary surgery. Breast. 2006;15(3):411-413.

(23) Kepics JM. Physical therapy treatment of axillary web syndrome. *Rehabil*

Oncol. 2004;22(1):21-22.

(24) Koehler LA. Treatment considerations for axillary web syndrome. Proceedings of the Seventh National Lymphedema Network International Conference, Nashville, TN; 25; November 2006.

(25) Cheville AL, Tchou J. Barriers to rehabilitation following surgery for primary breast cancer.J Surg Oncol. 2007;95(5):409-418.

(26) Fourie WJ, Robb KA. Physiotherapy management of axillary web syndrome following breast cancer treatment: discussing the use of soft tissue techniques.Physiotherapy. 2009;95(4):314-320.

(27) Wyrick SL, Waltke LJ, Ng AV. Physical therapy may promote resolution of lymphatic cording in breast cancer survivors.Rehabilitation Oncology. 2006;24(1):29-34.

(28) Torres Lacomba M, Mayoral Del Moral O, Coperias Zazo JL, Yuste Sanchez MJ, Ferrandez JC, Zapico Goni A. Axillary web syndrome after axillary dissection in breast cancer: a prospective study.Breast Cancer Res *Treat.* 2009;117(3):625-630.

(29) Koehler LA. Axillary Web Syndrome. Zuther, JE.Lymphedema Management, The Comprehensive Guide for Patients and Practitioners. 4th ed.New York, NY: Thieme Medical Scientific Publishers; 2009:70-72.

(30) Ridner SH, Dietrich MS, Stewart BR, Armer JM. FAAN. Body mass index and breast cancer treatment-related lymphedema. Support Care Cancer. 2011 Jun; 19(6): 853–857

(31) Helyer LK, Varnic RN, Le LW, Leong W, McCready D (2009) Obesity is a risk factor for developing postoperative lymphedema in breast cancer patients. Breast J16(1):48–54

(32) Greene AK, Grant FD, Slavin SA.Lower-extremity lymphedema and elevated body-mass index. N Engl J Med 2012; 366:2136-2137May 31, 2012DOI: 10.1056/NEJMc1201684

(33) Soran A, D'Angelo G, Begovic M, et al (2006) Breast cancer-related lymphedema – what are the significant predictors and how they affect the

severity of lymphedema? Breast J 12(6):536–43

(34) Farrow W. Phlebolymphedema–A Common Underdiagnosed and Undertreated Problem in the Wound Care Clinic.J Am Col Certif Wound Spec.2010; 2(1): 14–23. Published online 2010 Apr22.doi:10.1016/j.jcws.2010.04.004

(35) Pirard et al. The post-thrombotic syndrome - a condition to prevent .eScholarship,UC Davis.Dermatology Online Journal.Volume 14, Issue 3

(36) Herpertz, U. (1995) Das Lipödem. Lymphologie19, 1-11

(37) Kruppa P et al.Lipedema—Pathogenesis, Diagnosis, and Treatment Options.Dtsch Arztebl Int.2020 Jun; 117(22-23): 396–403.Published online 2020 Jun 1.doi:10.3238/arztebl.2020.0396

(38) Shin BW et al. Lipedema, A Rare Disease. Ann Rehabil Med.2011 Dec; 35(6): 922–927.Published online 2011 Dec 30.doi:10.5535/arm.2011.35.6.922

(39) Bertlich M et al. Lipedema in a male patient: report of a rare case – management and review of the literature.GMS Interdiscip Plast Reconstr Surg DGPW.2021; 10: Doc11.Published online 2021 Sep 22.doi:10.3205 iprs000161

(40) Child AH, Gordon KD, Sharpe P, Brice G, Ostergaard P, Jeffery S, Mortimer PS. Lipedema: an inherited condition. Am J Med Genet A. 2010;152A:970–976

(41) Herbst K et al. Standard of care for lipedema in the United States. Phlebology.2021 Dec; 36(10): 779–796. Published online 2021 May 28.doi:10.1177/02683555211015887

(42) Hassanein AH et al. Diagnostic Accuracy of Lymphoscintigraphy for Lymphedema and Analysis of False-Negative Tests. Plast Reconstr Surg GlobOpen.2017 Jul; 5(7): e1396. Published online 2017 Jul 12.doi:10.1097/GOX.0000000000001396

(43) Ridner SH et al.A Prospective Study of L-Dex Values in Breast Cancer Patients Pretreatment and Through 12 Months Postoperatively.Lymphatic Research and Biology. Vol16,No5.Published Online:16 Oct 2018https://doi.org/10.1089/lrb.2017.0070

(44) Fu M, Ridner SH, Hu SH, Cormier JC, Armer JM. Psychosocial impact of lymphedema: a systematic review of literature (2004–2011). Psycho-Oncology 2013; 22(7):1466-1484

(45) McWayne J, Heiney SP. Psychologic and social sequelae of secondary lymphedema: a review. Cancer 2005;104(3):457–466

(46) Ridner SH et al. Breast cancer treatment related lymphedema self-care; eduction, practices symptoms, and quality of life. Support Care Cancer, 2011; 19(5):631-637

(47) R.Ahmed et al. Lymphedema and Quality of Life in Breast Cancer Survivors: The Iowa Women's Health Study.J Clin Oncol. 2008 Dec 10; 26(35): 5689–5696. Published online 2008 Nov 10. doi:10.1200/JCO.2008.16.4731

(48) Greene A, Meskell P. The impact of lower limb chronic oedema on patients' quality of life. Int Wound J 2017; 14:561–568.

(49) Moffatt CJ, Aubeeluck A, Franks PJ, Doherty D, Mortimer P, Quere I. Psychological factors in chronic oedema: A case-control study. Lymphat Res Biol 2017; 15:252–260.

(50) Bowman C, Piedalue KA, Baydoun M, Carlson L. The Quality of Life and Psychosocial Implications of Cancer-Related Lower-Extremity Lymphedema: A Systematic Review of the Literature.J Clin Med.2020 Oct; 9(10): 3200. Published online 2020 Oct 2.doi:10.3390/jcm9103200

(51) Radina ME, Armer JM. Post-breast cancer lymphedema and the family: A qualitative investigation of families coping with chronic illness. J Fam Nurs 2001;7(3):281–299.

(52) Radina ME, Armer JM. Surviving breast cancer and living with lymphedema: resiliency among women in the context of their families. J Fam Nurs 2004;10(4):485–505

(53) Mirolo BR, Bunce IH, Chapman M, et al: Psychosocial benefits of postmastectomy lymphedema therapy. Cancer Nurs 18:197-205, 1995

3.0 Treatment of Lymphedema

At this time there is no cure for lymphedema; however, the symptoms associated with this condition can be often drastically mitigated with appropriate treatment. Successful therapy of lymphedema is ideally achieved by a multi-professional team effort between physicians with sufficient knowledge in the diagnosis and treatment of lymphedema, and well-trained and certified lymphedema therapists. Successful long-term treatment outcomes also requires the patient to be an active team member.

Despite recent advancements in the surgical approach for lymphedema (see 3.4), there is a broad consensus in the medical field that surgical modalities do not eliminate the need for non-surgical, conservative treatment for lymphedema achieved by a treatment modality known as Complete Decongestive Therapy (CDT), which is the first line gold-standard of care for this condition[1-3].

Newer generation intermittent pneumatic compression pumps can serve as a useful adjunct treatment to CDT, especially for lymphedema patients with limited or no access to medical care (see 3.3).

3.1 Lymphedema Therapists

Complete Decongestive Therapy is performed by certified lymphedema therapists. Several schools in the United States[4] offer specialized training and certification to physical, occupational and massage therapists, physicians, chiropractors, or nurses. Therapists attending these courses receive a minimum of 135 hours of specific lymphedema training, which consists of one third class room lecture and two thirds of lab instruction in order to learn the necessary skills to effectively treat lymphedema. Upon successful completion of a 135-hour course, which includes a written and hands-on examination, the participants graduate as certified lymphedema therapists (CLT). Unfortunately, at the current time there are no mandatory training standards for lymphedema therapists, and some health care professionals claim to be lymphedema therapists, but have not actually attended one of these nationally recognized 135-hour programs.

Lymphedema patients have been mistreated for hundreds of years and members of the lymphedema community, including patient advocates, therapists and educators have worked tirelessly over the past decades to improve treatment standards, while establishing meaningful and necessary guidelines for the training of lymphedema therapists in the US, Canada and worldwide.

The lack of standardized qualifications and training can seriously affect the outcome of lymphedema treatment, and patients should make sure that the lymphedema therapist of their choosing has attended and successfully graduated from a recognized lymphedema treatment program that offers in classroom (not *virtual*) hands-on instruction in the treatment techniques involved in CDT.

Recognized lymphedema training schools, as well as other sources, such as the National Lymphedema Network, or Lymphedema Blog, offer therapist resources on their websites, which enables patients to locate a certified therapist in their area[(4)].

3.2 Complete Decongestive Therapy

Complete Decongestive Therapy (CDT), also described as complex decongestive therapy or combined physical therapy, is a non-invasive and multi component treatment approach to lymphedema and related conditions, such as lipo-lymphedema and phlebo-lymphedema. Numerous studies have proven the scientific basis and effectiveness of this therapy[(2,5-7)], which has been established in European countries since the 1970s and has been practiced in the Americas in one form or another since the 1980s. CDT consists of a combination of treatment modalities that include manual lymph drainage (MLD), compression therapy with specialized bandage materials and garments, patient-tailored exercises and skin care.

The goal of CDT is to reduce lymphedema to a normal, or near normal size and to maintain this reduction, that is to prevent the re-accumulation of fluid in the tissues. Furthermore, lymphedema therapy aims to reduce fibrotic tissues associated with long-standing lymphedema, and to prevent infections (see 2.6.1).

In order to reduce the swelling with CDT, it is necessary to re-route the lymph flow and the excess protein and water molecules around the blocked areas into more centrally located healthy lymph vessels and lymph nodes in secondary lymphedema, and to identify and mobilize alternative and sufficient drainage pathways in primary cases.

3.2.1 Components of Complete Decongestive Therapy

Manual Lymph Drainage

Manual lymph drainage (MLD) is a manual treatment technique, which in most cases is applied with light pressure, and is based on four strokes, initially developed in the 1930s by Dr. Emil Vodder, a PhD. from Denmark.

These basic strokes are known as the *stationary circle*, *pump*, *rotary,* and *scoop* techniques, and are designed to manipulate lymph nodes and lymphatic vessels with the goal of increasing their activity and promoting the flow of lymph. In cases where hardened fibrotic tissues are present, which is often the case in long-standing chronic upper and lower extremity lymphedema, the pressure applied to the MLD strokes may be higher to manipulate lymph flow, depending on each individual case.

The common denominator of all strokes is the resting and working phase. In the working phase of the stroke, lymphatic structures located in the fatty tissues of the skin are stretched, resulting in an increase in their activity. In addition to increased lymphatic activity, the light directional pressure in the working phase of the strokes causes lymphatic fluid to move in the desired direction, thus contributing to the reduction of the swelling.

Certain MLD strokes are designed to manipulate lymph vessels located in the subcutaneous tissues of larger body surfaces, such as the trunk, other techniques are better suited to be applied on contoured surfaces, such as the extremities.

Stationary Circle: This technique consists of an oval-shaped stretching of the skin with the palmar surfaces of the fingers or the entire hand. Stationary circles can be applied with one hand, or both, and are used on the entire surface of the body, but mainly on lymph node groups (axilla and groin), the neck, and the face.

Pump technique: The entire palm and the proximal (upper) palmar surfaces of the fingers are used to apply a circle-shaped pressure on the skin, operating within almost the full range of motion in the therapist's wrist. Pump strokes are primarily used to manipulate lymph vessels located in the extremities and can be applied with one hand or both, in which case the hands move alternately.

Rotary technique: This technique is used on large body surface areas, such as the trunk. The entire palmar surface of the hand and fingers are used in an elliptical movement during the working phase. Like the scoop technique, rotaries are applied dynamically, meaning the working hand moves over the surface of the treated body part in a continuous fashion. If applied with both hands, the techniques are alternating.

Scoop technique: Scoops are applied mainly on the lower parts of extremities and consist of a spiral-shaped movement. During the working phase, which can be applied with one, or both alternating hands, the palmar surface of the hand moves dynamically over the skin. The hand movement is facilitated by transitional movement in the wrist, combined with forearm pronation and supination.

Compared to traditional massage, the pressure applied with manual lymph drainage is much lower in intensity. The goal of these techniques is to manipulate the lymphatic structures located in the tissues directly below the skin. In order to achieve the desired effect, the pressure in the working phase should be sufficient to mobilize the subcutaneous tissues against the fascia (a structure separating the skin from the muscle layer) located underneath, but not to manipulate the underlying muscle tissue.

In the resting phase of the stroke, the pressure is released, which supports the absorption of lymph fluid into lymph vessels. To achieve the maximum effect with each technique, the working phase with every stroke should last about one second and should be repeated five to seven times.

The overall goal of MLD in the treatment of lymphedema is to re-route the flow of stagnated lymphatic fluid around blocked areas into more centrally located healthy lymphatic vessels, which eventually drain into the venous system.

In the case of upper extremity lymphedema caused by breast cancer surgery, it is necessary to re-route the flow of stagnated lymph in the subcutaneous tissues of the arm around the blocked axillary area where the lymph nodes were removed, towards and into the axillary lymph nodes located on the opposite side, and the inguinal lymph nodes on the same side the surgery was performed. These groups of lymph nodes represent the drainage areas for the stagnant lymph fluid located in the affected upper extremity and need to be manipulated prior to initiating the treatment of the arm itself.

In the case of primary and secondary lower extremity lymphedema, the stagnated lymphatic fluid is generally re-routed around the blocked inguinal (groin) area towards and into the inguinal lymph nodes of the opposite side and the axillary lymph nodes on the same side of the blockage. As with lymphedema affecting the upper extremity, these groups of lymph nodes represent the drainage area for the stagnated lymph fluid and need to be manipulated prior to starting treatment of the leg.

The manipulation of these drainage areas with MLD strokes creates a "suction effect" in the healthy lymph vessels located in the drainage areas, which enables accumulated lymph fluid to move from a region with insufficient lymphatic drainage into an area with normal lymphatic drainage, and eventually back into the venous system.

Following this preparation, the extremity itself is treated in segments; the proximal (upper) aspect of the affected extremity is decongested prior to expanding the treatment to the more distal (lower) aspect of the arm or leg. This segmented approach ensures that lymph vessels located in more proximal areas of the extremity are properly prepared to handle incoming lymphatic fluid from areas located more distally.

In order to prevent re-accumulation of the fluid evacuated from the extremity, it is necessary that the MLD treatment is followed up with compression, which, depending on the stage of treatment, is applied either with specialized padded bandages or compression garments.

Manual lymph drainage presents a unique opportunity for health care professionals to specialize and opens the door to treating and manipulating a variety of conditions associated with dysfunctions of the lymphatic system. However, the unique techniques of manual lymph drainage deviate considerably from traditional manual techniques and therefore require specialized training in recognized schools.

Compression Therapy

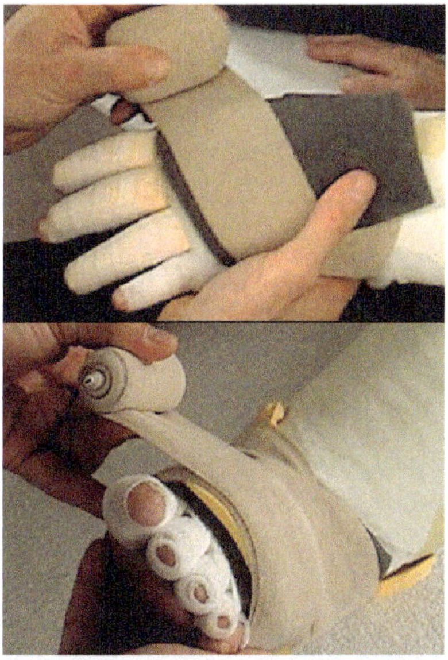

Fig. 3.1 Application of padded short-stretch compression bandages with foam pieces on the hand and foot. From Zuther J, Norton S Lymphedema Management, 4th ed. Thieme Publishers Stuttgart /New York (reprinted with permission)

Compression therapy in the treatment of lymphedema is applied by padded short-stretch bandages (Fig. 3.1), compression garments (Fig. 3.2), or alternative materials, such as adjustable compression devices (Fig. 3.3), and is an integral part of lymphedema management. The goal of compression therapy is to maintain and improve the reduction of the swelling achieved during lymphedema treatments.

It is important to understand that although the swelling in lymphedema may be reduced to a normal or near normal size during CDT treatments, the damage to the lymphatic system caused by the onset of lymphedema is permanent. In addition to the underlying damage to the lymphatic system, the elastic fibers in the tissues affected by lymphedema are damaged as well. These fibers loose their elasticity and tend to harden, especially in long-standing and untreated lymphedema present over a long period of time.

Without proper long-term management, the evacuated fluid, in most cases, will re-accumulate in the affected body part without compression. Contrary to edema, a low-protein swelling, lymphedema is a disease rather than a symptom and its underlying cause, the malfunction of parts of the lymphatic system, cannot be reversed. Compression bandages and garments by themselves will not reduce existing swelling and must therefore not be worn on an untreated, swollen extremity.

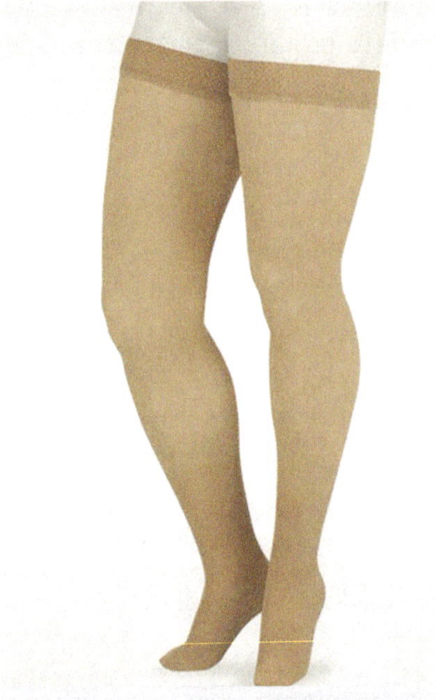

Fig. 3.2 Lower extremity garment with silicone border. With permission from JUZO USA, Inc.

Individuals affected by lymphedema graduate from padded short stretch bandages, which are applied by the lymphedema therapist in the intensive phase of CDT (see 3.2.2) to elastic compression garments only when the affected extremity is decongested.

To assist in the movement of fluids back to the heart, a pressure gradient between the lower (higher pressure) and the upper part (lower pressure) of the extremity is provided with bandages and garments.

Even after successful treatment, the body part affected by lymphedema is at permanent risk of repeat fluid build-up, and most individuals affected by lymphedema know that lymphedema condition requires life-long care.

Without the benefits of external compression, successful long-term management of lymphedema would be very difficult and, in most cases, impossible.

The application of external compression provides the necessary support for those tissues that lost elasticity, and compensates for the elastic insufficiency by increasing the tissue pressure.

The tissue pressure plays an essential role in the exchange of fluids between the blood capillaries and the tissue. The increased tissue pressure provided by external compression reduces the amount of fluid leaving the blood capillaries into the tissues, and increases the return of tissue fluids back into the blood and lymph capillaries, thus reducing the amount of fluid in the tissues.

External compression also increases venous and lymphatic return by improving the function of the valves within these vessels.

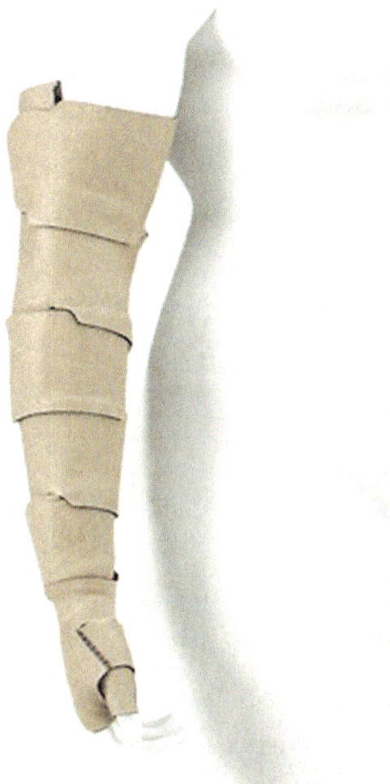

Fig. 3.3 Alternative compression with adjustable velcro straps. With permission from JUZO USA, Inc.

Another important factor for sufficient return of venous and lymphatic fluids back into the blood stream is the movement of skeletal musculature and joints during activity. Together with other supporting mechanisms, the muscle and joint pump activity propels these fluids back to the heart and ensures uninterrupted circulation.

External compression provides a counter force to the working musculature, known as working pressure, thus improving its efficiency.

These effects help to prevent re-accumulation of fluids evacuated during CDT treatments, and conserve the results achieved during MLD.

Another positive impact of compression therapy is the softening of hardened connective tissue, which is often present in lymphedema, especially if external compression therapy is combined with special foam materials (Fig. 3.1).

Compression Bandages

Compression bandages are used during the decongestive (intensive) phase of CDT (see 3.2.2). In this sequence of the treatment, the volume of the affected limb changes almost daily, and it is necessary that external compression adapts to these changes. Bandages are much better suited for this task than compression garments, such as sleeves and stockings, which would have to be re-fitted constantly in order to accommodate the changing volume of the affected extremity. Garments are used in the second phase of complete decongestive therapy when the limb is decongested, and changes in volume are minimal.

Crucial in lymphedema management is to provide the skin tissues with a solid counter force against the muscles working underneath, particularly while standing, sitting, walking, or performing therapeutic exercises. The subsequent increase in the tissue pressure during muscle activity promotes lymphatic and venous return and prevents fluid from accumulating in the skin. It is equally important to prevent the bandages from exerting too much pressure on the tissues during rest, which could cause a tourniquet effect and effectively prevent an adequate return of these fluids.

There are two distinct types of compression bandages; short-stretch and long-stretch bandages. The difference refers to the extent the bandages can be stretched from their original length. Short-stretch bandages are made from cotton fibers, which are interwoven in a way that allows for about 60% extensibility of its original length, whereas long-stretch bandages, commonly known as "ACE" bandages contain polyurethane, which allows for extensibility of more than 140% of the bandages' original length.

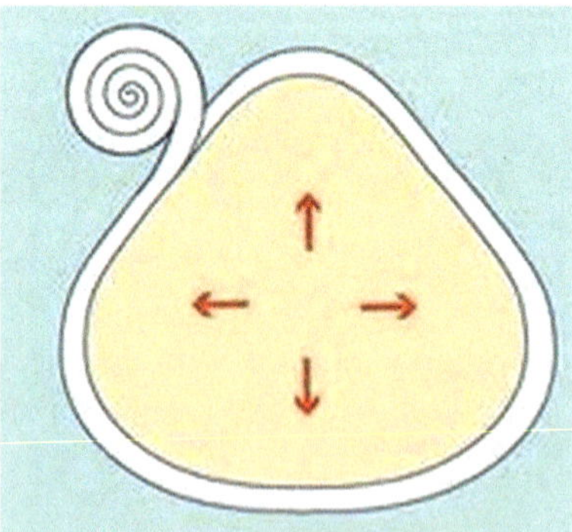

Fig. 3.4 Working pressure of short-stretch compression bandages

The extent to which a bandage can be stretched specifies the two main qualities of pressure in compression therapy, the working pressure and the resting pressure. The working pressure is determined by the resistance the bandage provides against the musculature working underneath, and is active only during muscle activity, and therefore temporary. The pressure the bandage exerts on the tissues at rest, that is without muscle contraction is known as the resting pressure, which is permanent. Relevant to these pressure qualities are the number of bandage layers, the tension with which these layers are applied, and most importantly, the type of bandage used.

The high working pressure of short-stretch cotton bandages provides the necessary solid counter force and makes them the preferred compression bandage in the management of lymphedema. Due to the low resting pressure of short-stretch bandages, tourniquet effects are prevented, provided these bandages are applied correctly.

Long-stretch ("ACE") bandages have the exact opposite effect and are not suitable for lymphedema management. The low working pressure these bandages provide does not offer adequate resistance, and fluid would inevitably accumulate. In addition, the high resting pressure of long-stretch bandages could constrict veins and lymph vessels during rest.

Prior to the application short-stretch bandages, appropriate skin moisturizers are applied, which is followed by tubular gauze to protect the bandages from the moisturizing lotions or creams; on top of the gauze special padding bandages, or foam materials are applied to distribute the pressure more evenly, and to prevent a tourniquet effect (Fig. 3.1).

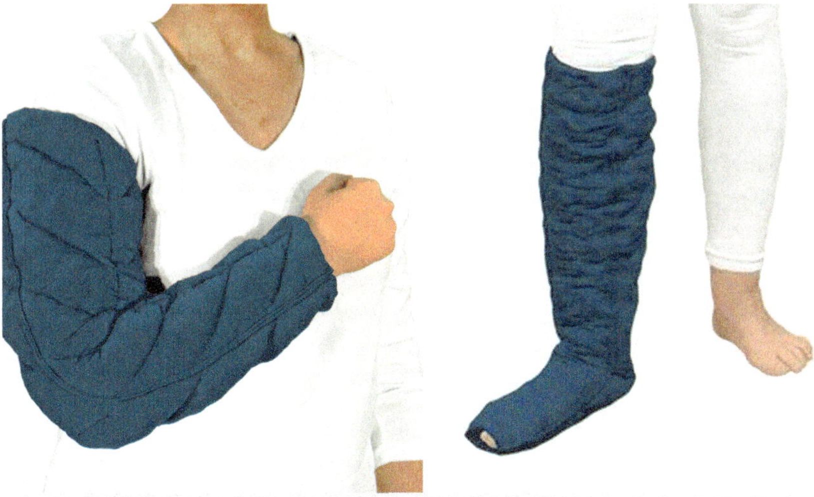

Fig. 3.5 (a), (b) Bandage liner for the arm and lower leg. With permission from Lohmann & Rauscher, USA Inc.

Padding can also be achieved with the combination of special bandage liners, which are applied underneath the short-stretch bandages. These liners are filled with foam particles and "built-in" channels to help direct the flow of lymph (Fig. 3.5 a, b); swell spots or pads, which are available in different shapes and sizes, and are filled with soft foam pieces, can be used underneath compression bandages for added compression in localized swelling, or to protect bony prominences. Pads are also available to accommodate swelling affecting the genital areas.

Compression Garments

While compression in the first, or intensive phase of CDT is applied by padded short-stretch bandages, patients graduate to compression garments once the extremity is decongested to a normal or near-normal size in the second phase of treatment. Patients are fitted for garments directly following the intensive phase of CDT by someone who is experienced, or certified in taking measurements for compression garments, such as certified lymphedema therapists or certified garment fitters.

The primary goal of compression garments is to maintain the reduction achieved during the intensive phase of CDT; it is important to understand that compression garments are not designed to be worn at night time, or to further reduce lymphedema, and should only be worn on a decongested extremity.

Compression garments for extremities such as sleeves, gauntlets, stockings and pantyhose, or those manufactured for other parts of the body, such as vests and brassieres, are available in several sizes, variations, and compression classes.

Selecting an appropriate compression garment is a challenging task, and many important factors, such coverage area, the general shape of the limb, mobility and activity level, age, compression class, material, cost, skin sensitivity and integrity, the possible presence of arterial diseases and donning/doffing issues need to be considered. Some of these factors play a major role in the process to determine if a custom-made or ready-made compression garment would be the better choice for the individual.

Styles and Variations

Custom made-to-measure garments, or standard size, also labeled as over-the-counter (OTC) garments, can be ordered in various compression classes, styles, colors, patterns and lengths, as well as fastening systems, such as hip attachments, shoulder straps, or borders that prevent sliding of the garment. (Figs. 3.6 to 3.9).

Fig. 3.6 (a) glove (b) gauntlet. With permission from JUZO USA, Inc

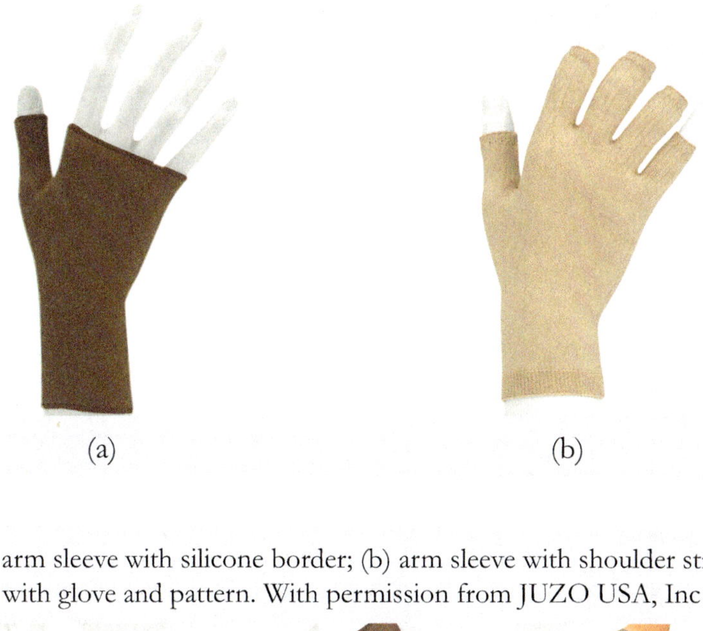

(a) (b)

Fig. 3.7 (a) arm sleeve with silicone border; (b) arm sleeve with shoulder strap; (c) arm sleeve with glove and pattern. With permission from JUZO USA, Inc

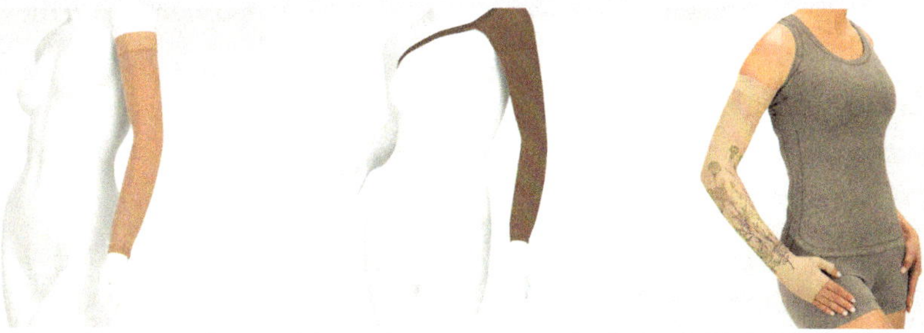

(a) (b) (c)

Fig. 3.8 (a) foot with toes; (b) knee high with foot and toes; (c) knee high with silicone border. With permission from JUZO USA, Inc.

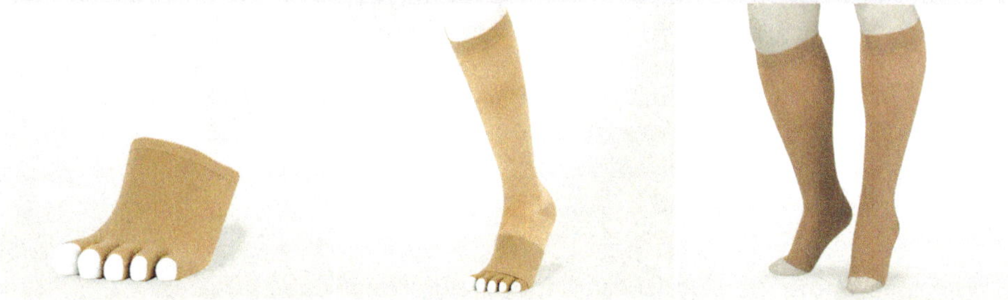

(a) (b) (c)

Fig. 3.9 (a) thigh high with silicone border; (b) thigh high with hip attachment; (c) pantyhose. With permission from JUZO USA, Inc.

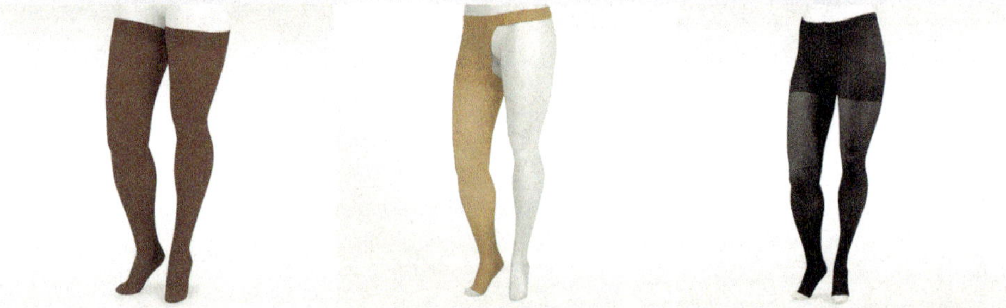

(a) (b) (c)

It is important that the garments are applied correctly and without any creases or folds over the length of the extremity, and that the garment reaches all the way up to the axilla or groin to prevent fluid build-up close to the root of the extremity. Donning and doffing aids, which are available from a number of garment manufacturers, as well as rubber donning gloves assist in the application, and protect garment damage from finger nails or jewelry.

Alternative Compression

For patients who may have difficulties in donning or doffing compression garments, or are unable to apply bandages, have very irregular shaped limbs, or just wish to use an alternative compression product, there are a number of devices available that provide gradient compression. These devices are easy to put on and can be adjusted for fluctuations in shape and size using non-elastic and adjustable bands with hook and loop closures. Alternative compression materials are applied on top of liners and padding, which protect the skin, and the product from moisturizers. These devices, or wraps require the measurements be taken by the lymphedema therapist or certified fitter, and can also be used in venous caused swellings and wound care, as well as other conditions (Figs. 3.10, 3.11).

Fig. 3.10 (a) hand wrap; (b) hand and arm wrap; (c) foot and full leg wrap. With permission from JUZO USA, Inc.

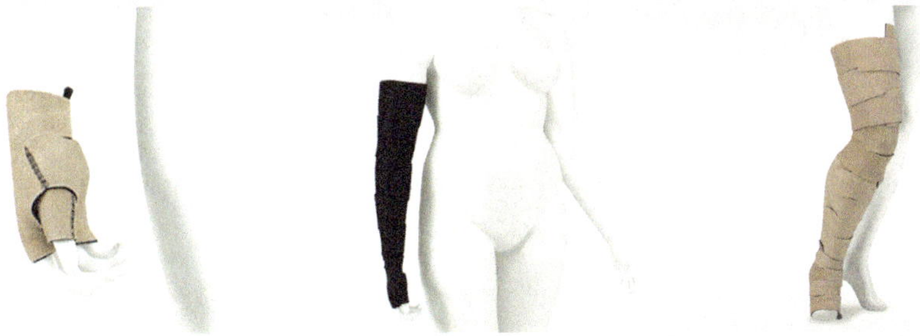

(a) (b) (c)

Fig. 3.11 (a) calf wrap with liner; (b) foot wrap; (c) foot and full leg wrap with hip attachment. With permission from JUZO USA, Inc.

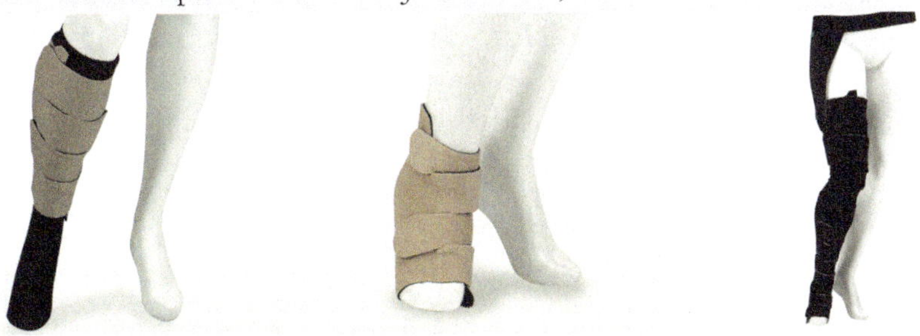

(a) (b) (c)

Compression Classes

Compression garments for extremities are available in several compression classes, or levels. The level of compression within the different classes is determined by the value of pressure the garments produce on the surface of the skin; these pressure values are measured in units of millimetres of mercury (mmHg), a measure of pressure also used to compute blood pressure. Compression classes are specified by a range of numbers, such as 30-40 mm/Hg, which indicates that the level, or amount of pressure produced on the surface of the skin will not exceed 40 mm/Hg, or fall below 30 mm/Hg.

For a compression garment to work effectively and to not produce a stagnation of fluid, or a tourniquet effect, the pressure needs to gradually decrease from the lower part to the upper portion of an extremity. This graduated compression ensures that pressure is highest on the ankle and wrist, and lowest at the shoulder and hip.

Most manufacturers use the following pressure values within the compression classes, which range from 1 to 4; seamed, or custom garments (values indicated in brackets) are available in all classes, seamless, or over-the-counter garments are available in classes 1 to 3:

- Class 1: 20-30 mm/Hg for seamless garments (18-21 seamed)
- Class 2: 30-40 mm/Hg for seamless garments (23-32 seamed)
- Class 3: 40-50 mm/Hg for seamless garments (34-46 seamed)
- Class 4: more than 50 mm/Hg

In general, compression levels provided by class 2 garments will be sufficient to prevent swelling in most patients affected by lymphedema of the upper extremity; patients with involvement of the leg will in most cases require a garment with compression class 3.

However, there are several exceptions to this general rule; some patients with lower extremity lymphedema may require garments with lower compression levels than those provided in class 3, or maybe a garment of higher compression. Alternatively, patients with lymphedema of the arm may use a compression class 1 sleeve, or even class 3 in some cases.

Many factors must be considered by the physician and/or lymphedema therapist to determine the correct compression class for each individual patient. Tolerance to external compression, age, physical limitations, activity level, skin integrity, and possible additional conditions, such as arterial insufficiencies, pareses or paralysis, or cardiac issues may influence the choice of compression class.

Compression levels below 20 mm/Hg, which falls in the support stocking category, are not sufficient for lymphedema management. These support, or anti-embolism socks, generally available in big box stores, may be less expensive than compression garments, and provide some support that can be sufficient for swellings following minor injuries, such as sprains. However, they don't come close to providing the support necessary to maintain the swelling associated with lymphedema, which requires medical grade compression.

Ineffective compression results in further complications and often results in frustration on the patients' side, reducing compliance.

Patients receiving the advice from a health care provider to purchase an ineffective support garment versus a compression garment specifically geared towards the management of lymphedema should immediately terminate this relationship and seek consultation from a properly trained and certified lymphedema therapist. A health care provider familiar with the pathology of lymphedema would never recommend ineffective support garments for the management of lymphedema.

Custom and Ready-Made Garments

Compression garments are manufactured using an inlay thread generally made of Lycra or a rubber material, which provides a high level of compression consistency; these threads are covered with cotton or a synthetic material. Both custom and ready-made garments used in lymphedema therapy contain this thread, which is woven into the material in a continuous manner. The different compression levels are achieved by adjusting the tension of this inlay thread.

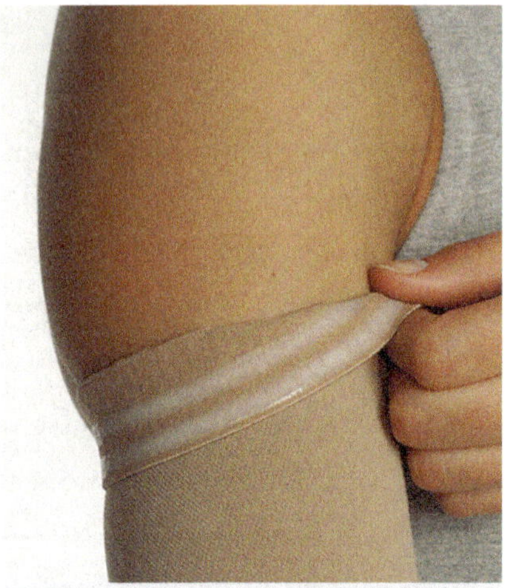

Fig. 3.12 Silicone border on an arm sleeve. With permission from JUZO USA, Inc.

Ready-made, or over-the-counter (OTC) garments are made from relatively thin and sheer fabrics that are continually knitted in a circular fashion on a cylinder and have no seam. The appropriate shape and size of the garment is created by varying stitch height and yarn tension. Generally, these garments tend to be more cosmetically appealing and lighter in weight. Ready-made garments are less expensive, easier to replace, and quicker to obtain than custom-made garments, and come in a variety of girths, lengths, and fabrics.

The disadvantages of ready-made garments are that they may not provide enough support and are not as precise in fit like a garment, which is custom-made to the individuals' exact measurements. They also tend to roll at the top if a silicone border is not added on the inside of the upper part (Fig. 3.12).

Custom-made compression garments are generally made from thicker, but breathable materials, and knitted row by row as a flat piece, which is shaped and produced by adding or removing needles during the production process, according to the exact measurements of the patient. The flat piece is then joined by a seam to form the garment. Custom garments can be made to fit any shape and are available in all four compression classes. The heavier knit materials provide greater stiffness resulting in greater resistance and better containment of the swelling than ready-made garments. There are several factors that determine the choice between a custom and ready-made garment.

Shape: although ready-made garments are available in a variety of sizes from most manufacturers, they are generally made for limbs of average proportion and length. Although some ready-made garments allow for an extra wide calf, elbow, thigh, or upper arm, a patient with a distorted or disproportionate limb will generally require a custom-made garment. Even if the individual circumferential measurements fall within the range of a specific ready-made garment size, some patients may have a disproportionate large calf, with measurements at the top end of the range and a relatively thin ankle with measurements on the low end of the range. The result would be a looser fit around the ankle area, which could result in a tourniquet effect with fluid accumulating in the ankle area.

For heavier patients, custom-made garments are often the only available option; however, some ready-made pregnancy garments, which can be obtained at a lower cost, may accommodate the measurements of these individuals.

Compression classes: Ready-made garments are available in compression classes 1 through 3, and custom garments are available in all four compression levels. The highest level, compression class 4, is reserved for the more severe and challenging cases of lymphedema.

Given the high compression of these garments, it is important that the ankle-brachial index (ABI) of the individual is tested by a health care professional. The ABI compares the blood pressure of the ankle to that of the arm and is used to determine if peripheral arterial disease (PAD) is present. While an ABI index of less than 0.5 presents a general contraindication for compression therapy, the ABI should be greater than 0.8 if a compression class 4 garment is prescribed.

A normal resting ankle-brachial index ranges between 0.9 and 1.3, which means that the blood pressure in the ankle area is the same or greater than the pressure in the arm.

Donning issues: some patients may have difficulty in donning a garment, especially a compression class 4 garment. In these cases, it is possible to layer two garments of lesser compression, for example, two compression class 1 garments on top of each other can be used to achieve up to 40 mm/Hg pressure. With the first garment applying 20-30 mm/Hg, the second garment will add about two-thirds of the pressure applied by the first garment. The layering of two compression garments also increases the stiffness factor, which results in greater resistance and better containment.

Skin integrity: if wounds or other skin conditions are present, it may be better to go with a more breathable custom garment. In some cases, it may be necessary to apply an under-stocking made of silk or cotton to avoid slippage of wound dressings while donning the garment. Compression garments containing silver may present a good option; silver threads woven into the garment have natural antimicrobial properties, prevent odor, and are commonly used in the treatment of wounds. In some cases, a zipper option may be considered if wounds are present.

Cosmetics: the appearance of a garment is very important to many patients. In some cases, it may be necessary to choose a less desirable option to further patient compliance. It is important to understand that there is no therapeutic value in a compression garment that is not worn by the patient for cosmetic reasons.

Measurements for Ready-Made Garments

Most manufacturers provide various styles of ready-made compression sleeves and stockings in a variety of sizes, colors and patterns. Custom sleeves should be ordered if the extremity is either too large or too small for standard-size garments.

It is highly recommended that trained specialists with a thorough understanding of lymphedema take the measurements (lymphedema therapist or certified fitter) and teach patients how to wear them properly. However, it may be necessary that patients measure on their own if ready-made garment are acquired directly from an online retailer for example. If this is the case, the measurements should be taken by a friend, or spouse and the measurements should be written down on a notepad.

Ideally, the measurements should be taken when the extremity is at its most reduced state, and be done early in the morning when the arm or leg is smallest, at the end of a treatment, or after the compression bandages have been removed.

Sizing for medical compression garments is based on the circumferences at specific points, as well as the length of the extremity. Measurements are taken with a tape measure, which should be applied in a straight fashion; a twisted or crooked tape measure will result in inaccurate measurements. If a tape measure is unavailable, a string and a ruler may be used. The circumferential and length measurements can be taken with the string and the individual lengths of the string are then measured with the ruler.

It is recommended to mark the skin with a non-permanent, non-toxic marker at each circumferential measurement made. The individual circumferential measurements, as well as the length measurement are then compared with the sizing chart of the manufacturer of choice to determine size and length of the compression garment.

Measurements for Arm Sleeves

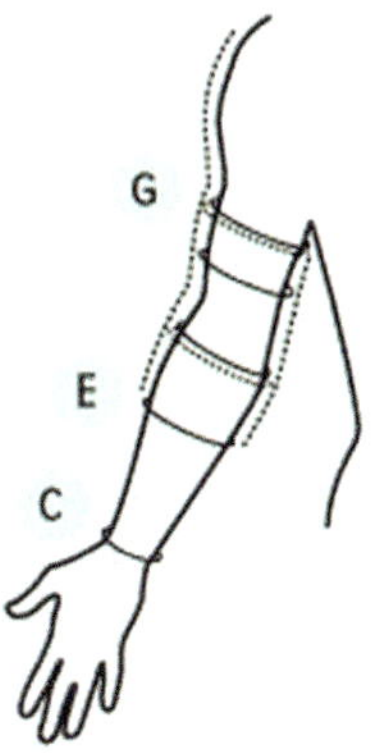

15-20, 20-30 and 30-40 mmHg

2000 / 2001 / 2002, 3511 / 3512

		I	II	III	IV	V	VI
G	Max	26.5-33 cm 10 1/2"-13"	28.5-35.0 cm 11 1/4"-13 3/4"	30.5-37.5 cm 12"-14 3/4"	32.5-39.5 cm 12 3/4"-15 1/2"	34.0-42.0 cm 13 1/2"-16 1/2"	36.0-44.0 cm 14 1/2"-17 1/2"
	Reg.	21.5-26 cm 8 1/2"-10 1/2"	23.5-28.5 cm 9 1/4"-11 1/4"	25.0-31.0 cm 9 3/4"-12 1/4"	27.0-33.0 cm 10 1/2"-13"	29.0-35.0 cm 11 1/2"-13 3/4"	30.5-37.5 cm 12"-14 3/4"
E	Max	22.5-27.5 cm 8 3/4"-10 3/4"	24.5-29.5 cm 9 3/4"-11 1/4"	26-32 cm 10 1/4"12 1/2"	27.5-33.5 cm 10 3/4"-13 1/4"	29.0-35.0 cm 11 1/2"-13 3/4"	30.0-37.0 cm 11 3/4"-14 1/2"
	Reg.	20.5-25.5 cm 8"-10"	22-27 cm 8 3/4"-10 3/4"	23.5-28.5 cm 9 1/4"-11 1/4"	25.0-30.0 cm 9 3/4"-11 3/4"	26.0-32.0 cm 10 1/4"-12 1/2"	27.5-33.5 cm 10 3/4"-13 1/4'
C	C	14.0-15.5 cm 5 1/2"-6"	15.5-17.0 cm 6"-6 3/4"	17.0-18.5 cm 6 3/4"-7 1/4"	18.5-20 cm 7 1/4"-7 3/4"	20.0-21.5 cm 7 3/4"-8 1/2"	21.5-23 cm 8 1/2"-9"

C-G/C-H Regular - C-G length < 17" / 43 cm   C-G/C-H Long - C-G length > 17" / 43 cm

Fig. 3.13 Measurement and sizing chart for arm sleeves. With permission from JUZO USA, Inc

C: Wrist Circumference

This is the point of greatest compression and therefore an important point. Place the measuring tape at the narrowest part of the wrist, at the transition from the hand to the forearm and measure the circumference. Find the smallest circumference at this measuring point. Write this measurement down and label it as a wrist measurement.

E: Elbow Circumference

Measure the largest part around the elbow with the arm slightly bent; the objective here is to get the largest measurement. Write this measurement down and label it as elbow measurement.

G: Upper Arm Circumference

This measurement is taken around the top of the upper arm in the axillary fold. To determine the correct location of this point, it is often helpful to place a book or something similar into the armpit area. The measuring point will be even with the top end of the book. Write this measurement down and label it as upper arm measurement.

C-G: Length Measurement

Measure the distance between the wrist circumference measuring point to the upper arm circumference point along the front of the arm. This measurement determines the length of your arm; write it down. You can now compare your measurements with the sizing chart of the manufacturer of your choice to determine the size and length of your sleeve. To do that, start with the measurement taken at the C-measurement around the wrist, and determine where that size fits into on the chart (Fig. 3.13). This measurement will determine the size of the garment. Example: if the measurement reads 17cm, it would fit in a size III; from now on you can ignore the other sizes and concentrate on size III and determine if the regular E-measurement around the elbow also fits in that size and continue to check the regular G-measurement. If the measurements all fall within size III, then your sleeve should be ordered in a regular size III.

Should the wrist measurement fall within size III, but the elbow and upper arm circumference measurements are somewhat larger, this manufacturer offers “Max” sizes to leave more room in these areas. In this case, a size III Max should be ordered. If the length measurement falls on 43cm or below, a regular length sleeve is appropriate, with lengths over 43cm a long sleeve should be ordered.

More measurements are needed if an additional compression gauntlet is required:

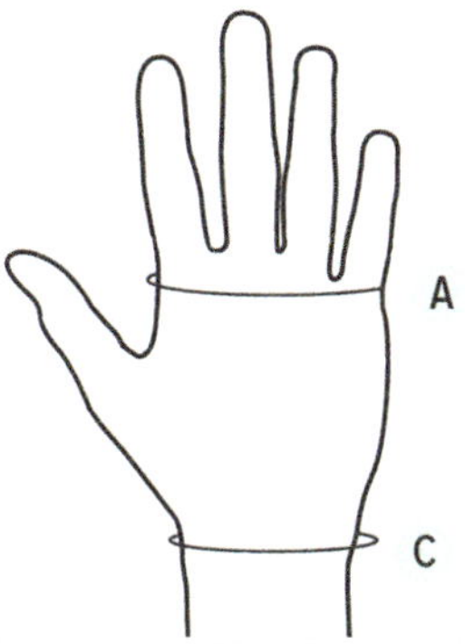

	S	M	L	XL
A	17.5-19.5 cm 6 7/8"-7 5/8"	19.5-21.0 cm 7 5/8"-8 1/4"	21.0-23.0 cm 8 1/4"-9 1/8"	23.0-25.5 cm 9 1/8"-10 1/8"
C	14.5-16.5 cm 5 5/8"-6 1/2"	16.5-18.0 cm 6 1/2"-7"	18.0-20.0 cm 7"-7 7/8"	20.0-22 cm 7 7/8"-8 5/8"

Fig. 3.14 Measurement and sizing chart for gauntlet. With permission from JUZO USA, Inc

C: Wrist Circumference

This is the same point measured for sleeves, and provides the highest compression; it is therefore an important point. Place the measuring tape at the narrowest part of the wrist, at the transition from the hand to the forearm and measure the circumference. Find the smallest circumference at this measuring point. Write this measurement down and label it as a wrist measurement.

A: Palm Circumference

Measure the width of the palm along the finger joints. Place the measuring tape around the palm with the palm up and the fingers slightly spread and measure the circumference. Write this measurement down and label it as a palm measurement.

Length measurements are not required for standard-sized compression gauntlets. You can now compare your measurements with the sizing chart of the manufacturer of your choice to determine the size of your gauntlet.

Measurements for Knee-High Stockings

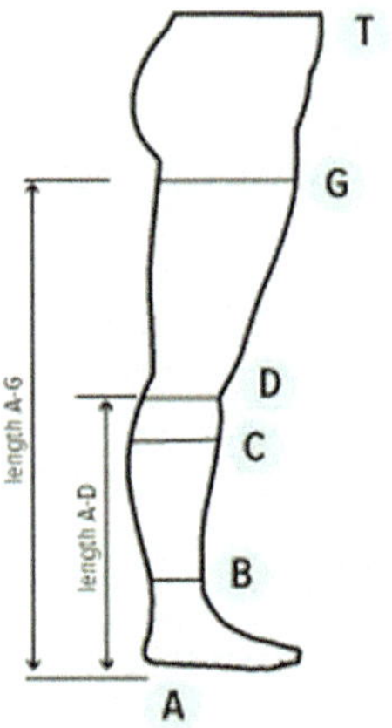

15-20, 20-30 and 30-40 mmHg

2100/01/02, 2000/2001/02, 2081/82, 3511/12, 3520/3521/3522, 2061/2062, 6091/6092

	I	II	III	IV	V
G	41-60 cm 16 1/4" - 23 1/2"	50-68 cm 19 1/2" - 26 3/4"	54-75 cm 21 1/4" - 29 1/2"	57-79 cm 22 1/2" - 31"	62-85 cm 24 1/2" - 33 1/2"
G	45-55 cm 17 3/4"- 21 1/2"	50-61 cm 19 1/2"- 24"	54-68 cm 21 1/4"- 26 3/4"	57-73 cm 22 1/2"- 28 3/4"	62-78 cm 24 1/2"- 30 3/4"
C	29-38 cm 11 1/2" - 15"	34-43 cm 13 1/4" - 17"	37-49 cm 14 1/2"-19 1/4"	41-53 cm 16 1/4" - 21"	46-58 cm 18" - 23"
B	18-21 cm 7" - 8 1/4"	21-24 cm 8 1/4" - 9 1/2"	24-27 cm 9 1/2"-10 3/4"	27-31 cm 10 3/4" - 12 1/4"	31-35 cm 12 1/4" - 13 3/4"

PCSZ-0102h

length A-D		length A-G	
A-D Regular	15 3/4-18 1/4" / 40-46 cm	A-G / AT Regular	28 1/4-32 3/4" / 72-83 cm
A-D Short	13-15 3/4" / 34-40 cm	A-G / AT Short	24 3/4-28 1/4" / 63-72 cm
A-D Petite	< 13" / 33 cm	A-G / AT Petite	21 3/4-24 3/4" / 55-63 cm

Fig. 3.15 Measurement and sizing chart for knee-high and thigh-high stockings. With permission from JUZO USA, Inc

B: Ankle Circumference

This is the area of greatest compression and therefore an important point. Place the measuring tape at the narrowest part of the ankle, just above the ankle bone, and measure the circumference. Write this measurement down and label it as ankle measurement.

C: Calf Circumference

Measure the largest part of the calf. You may need to search for the largest part of the calf by measuring above and below the middle of the calf; the objective here is to get the largest measurement. Write this measurement down and label it as calf measurement.

A-D: Length Measurement

Measure from the floor to the bend behind the knee; do not wear shoes as you will get an inaccurate measurement. Make sure that you are measuring just below the bend of the knee. Measuring too high or too close to the bend of the knee may result in a stocking too long for your lower leg, especially if your length measurement is right on the edge of the short and long length threshold, which is at the 40cm mark.

This measurement determines the length of your leg, write it down. You can now compare your measurements with the sizing chart of the manufacturer of your choice to determine the size and length of your stocking.

Knee-high compression stockings can be ordered in different lengths, with an open or closed-toe option and with or without a silicone border on the top to prevent sliding.

When you receive your stockings, it is important to put your stockings on first thing in the morning, right after the shower.

Measurements for Thigh-High Stockings

Refer to Fig. 3.15 for measurement and sizing. In addition to the ankle and calf measurements described under knee-high stockings, two additional measurements are necessary:

G: Thigh Circumference

Find the widest part of your thigh, right below your buttocks. Measure the circumference of this part of your thigh. Write this measurement down and label it as thigh measurement.

A-G: Length Measurement

For thigh high garments measure the length of leg from the top of the thigh, where the G-measurement was taken, to the floor behind the heel. This is the length of your leg, write it down on a notepad. You can now compare your measurements with the sizing chart for the brand of stockings you have chosen to determine the size and length of your stocking.

Thigh-high compression stockings can be ordered in different lengths, with an open or closed-toe option and with or without a silicone border on the top to prevent sliding.

When you receive your stockings, it is important to put your stockings on first thing in the morning, right after the shower.

Exercises

When a portion of the lymphatic system is injured by trauma, surgery, or radiation, or develops abnormally, the functionality of the lymphatic system is impaired, which can cause swelling most often affecting the upper or lower extremities.

A well-balanced exercise program in combination with other components of complete decongestive therapy used in the management of lymphedema plays an important part in reducing the swelling, and presents a vital tool for patients to continue with normal activities of daily living.

Patients who have lymphedema, or are at risk for developing it, profoundly benefit from regular exercises, which assists in weight control, decreased severity and prevention of lymphedema related symptoms, such as restricted joint mobility, and improves immune function, mood and energy level. Exercises also support venous and lymphatic return to the blood circulatory system, which assists decongestion and helps to maintain the reduction of lymphedema swelling achieved during the decongestive phase of treatment. An important factor to support and improve venous and lymphatic return is to wear the compression bandages or garments during exercise.

While the body of research is still limited, and most available studies focus on breast cancer related lymphedema (BCRL), there is ample evidence in support of the benefits of exercises in the management of lymphedema.

Lymphedema patients are often advised to protect their extremity from overuse following surgery, especially concerning resistive and aerobic exercises, which is certainly a valid advise; however, there is ample evidence that exercises are not linked to the worsening of lymphedema symptoms, and are beneficial if performed with slow progression in intensity and under initial supervision of a trained health care professional[8-11].

Patients are often unsure if they can continue their pre-lymphedema exercise activities, or if they should adjust, or replace them. The answer to that question depends on the kind of activity. For example, tennis or golf does not rank very high on the list of beneficial activities for individuals with upper extremity lymphedema, due to the risk of injury. For patients with lymphedema of the leg, kickboxing and step-aerobics are activities that bear a great risk of injury and should therefore be avoided.

However, for some individuals specific exercises play such a vital role in their daily routine that giving up these so-called "high-risk activities" would seriously impact their well-being.

These individuals should continue with their exercise regimen, even if it is tennis for patients with lymphedema of the arm, or running for those affected by lower extremity lymphedema. The fact is that nobody knows better than the lymphedema patient what is good for their body and spirit. If the patients are under the care of a trained lymphedema therapist, wear their compression garments or bandages during these physical activities, and the exercise regimen does not cause discomfort or pain, it is fine to continue with these activities.

However, if the affected limb hurts, feels strained, or increases in volume during and after the activity, the patient should adjust as necessary and consult with their lymphedema therapist or physician. The keywords here are caution and moderation; gradual progression is imperative while trying to accomplish an improved return of lymphatic fluid without adding further stress to an impaired lymphatic system.

Exercise protocols are customized by the lymphedema therapist and physician to meet individual goals for patients affected by lymphedema. The specific exercise protocols are determined by considering the stage and type of lymphedema, specific restrictions and limitations of joint and muscle activity, as well as additional medical conditions.

For most patients at risk of developing, or being diagnosed with lymphedema an exercise regimen typically includes some combination of flexibility and stretching exercises, resistive and aerobic exercises and breathing techniques.

More information on exercises for lymphedema is available in section 3.6.3.Self-Management of Lymphedema – Exercises.

Flexibility and Stretching Exercises

These exercises move the skin, muscle, and other tissues in the affected area, and assist in relieving the feeling of tightness that is often associated with lymphedema. An effective flexibility training program can also improve physical performance and help reduce the risk of injury. By improving the range of motion, the body requires less energy to make the same movements; it also contributes to more flexible joints and ligaments thus lessening the likelihood of injuries.

Mild Yoga may be especially helpful to promote both flexibility and relaxation.

Resistive Exercises

Resistive, or strength exercises improve muscular power, increase the strength in ligaments, tendons, and bones, and positively contribute to weight control; a high body-mass-index (BMI) is a well-known risk factor for lymphedema.

Resistive exercises are generally performed in a repetitive fashion against an opposing force, by using weights, resistance bands or ones own body weight. It is important to gradually increase strength training, and the exercise programs chosen should be appropriate to the patient's fitness level without adding further stress to an impaired lymphatic system. Certain strength exercises are beneficial for lymphedema patients and should always be performed with the compression garment or bandage in place. Resistive exercises using weights present possible problems regarding injury or overuse. However, with appropriate precautions resistive exercises using gradually increasing weights can be very beneficial(9).

An improved baseline of strength will allow daily tasks to be performed with less effort, can prevent overuse syndrome and restore muscular balance and normal bio-mechanics to the involved limb and surrounding joints. When beginning a resistance program, weights should be light, with higher repetitions, as opposed to choosing the heaviest weight the patient can only lift 1-3 times. Negative effects in terms of accumulation of fluid in the affected limb, or the limb at risk, are unlikely if exercises are performed with compression in place on the involved extremity.

Aerobic Exercises

Aerobic conditioning is generally performed in a repetitive fashion using large muscle groups. Some long-term benefits include a decrease in resting heart rate, improved muscular strength, weight control, and increased return of venous and lymphatic fluids. Aerobic exercises assist in weight loss and encourage deep breathing, which in turn supports lymphatic and venous return.

Beneficial activities for upper and lower extremity lymphedema include:

Swimming/Water Aerobics: With the body weight reduced by about 90% in chest-deep water, exercises performed in the water improve mobility and enhances strength and muscle tone. In addition, the pressure exerted by the water on the body surface contributes to lymphatic and venous return. Hot water with temperatures above 94 degrees F, usually found in hot tubs and Jacuzzis, should be avoided. High water temperature has a negative impact on lymphedema.

Walking: A 20-minute walk outdoors, or on a treadmill for 10-15 minutes and slow walking speed while wearing the compression garment, stimulates the circulatory system and contributes to general well-being. Key points: walk with a normal gait; do not drag the affected leg and avoid limping.

Easy Biking: 25-20 minutes either outdoors or at the gym, using a comfortable and wide saddle. Legs are placed in a higher position on recumbent bikes, which makes them a better choice for individuals affected by lower extremity lymphedema.

Yoga: The combination of stretching, deep breathing, relaxation, and the positive impact on the venous and lymphatic return, makes yoga a perfect choice of exercise. Strenuous yoga practices should be avoided, and if certain poses seem uncomfortable, they should be altered, or skipped. Many cancer centers and support groups have contacts for yoga classes specifically tailored to cancer survivors and lymphedema patients

Decongestive Exercises: The exercise program practiced with the lymphedema therapist during the intensive phase of complete decongestive therapy is tailored to each individual patient's needs, abilities and restrictions. This exercise regimen, which should ideally be performed twice daily, improves circulation, mobility, and well-being.

In general, exercises and activities should always be performed with the compression garment in place; an older compression garment can be used for exercises in the water. Intensity and duration of any exercise should be gradually increased, and movements that over-strain, cause discomfort or pain should be avoided.

Breathing Exercises

The downward and upward movement of the diaphragm in deep abdominal breathing is an essential component for the sufficient return of lymphatic fluid back to the bloodstream. Patients affected by lymphedema of the leg benefit greatly from an exercise program including diaphragmatic breathing exercises.

Abdominal breathing exercises are also beneficial for patients affected by lymphedema of the arm. The movement of the diaphragm, combined with the outward and inward movements of the abdomen, rib cage, and lower back, also promotes general well-being, peristalsis and return of venous blood back to the heart.

General rules on exercising with lymphedema:

Use common sense: Lifting heavy weights or running a marathon is not the best way to start a lymphedema exercise regimen. An exercise program should start gradually to avoid sprains and injury to muscles and should be followed by a warm down after active exercises. Studies have shown that a 10–15-minute warming down assists the lymphatic system in the removal of excess fluid and metabolites, which have accumulated in the tissues.

Observe: Watch your extremity during and after exercise activity for any change in comfort level, size, shape, texture, heaviness, or firmness. Any changes could be an indication that you need to adjust a particular activity or take a break. If a change persists for more than a few days, consult with your doctor or lymphedema therapist.

Use available resources: Work with a lymphedema therapist or other health care professional with knowledge in the treatment of lymphedema. At the beginning of an exercise regimen, it is beneficial to work with someone with expertise in lymphedema management who can provide valuable guidance and feedback. In many cases, the exercise program is individualized to take into consideration the stage of lymphedema, possible accompanying medical conditions, such as heart problems, pulmonary issues, diabetes, etc, or if you are taking any medication that has side effects.

Once you are familiar with the exercise program, you will be able to work on your own. If, for any reason, you do not have access to a lymphedema therapist or a health care professional with knowledge in lymphedema, consult with a Physical Therapist and explain your specific situation. These professionals have access to information specific to lymphedema and will be able to provide guidance.

Working with instructors and trainers without a medical background and no knowledge of the specific issues regarding lymphedema may have adverse effects, such as increased swelling or injury.

Skin Care

Skin and nail care play an essential role in the prevention of lymphedema in those patients who are at risk of developing this condition, and in the management of existing lymphedema.

The skin is the first line of defense against foreign invaders and is usually impermeable to pathogens. However, any defect in the skin such as burns, chafing, dryness, cuticle injury, cracks, cuts, splinters, insect bites, and tattoo needles can present an entry site for bacteria and cause infection.

Tissues affected by lymphedema are saturated with fluid rich in protein, which serves as an ideal nutrient source for bacteria and other pathogens. The skin in lymphedema tends to be dry and may become thickened and scaly, thereby increasing the risk of skin cracks and fissures.

The processes involved in inflammation not only worsen lymphedema by increasing the swelling, but can also develop into a medical crisis. The basic consideration in skin and nail care is therefore the prevention and control of infections, which includes proper cleansing and moisturizing techniques with the goal of maintaining the health and integrity of the skin.

Suitable ointments or lotions formulated for sensitive skin and lymphedema should be applied before the application of lymphedema bandages while the patient is in the intensive phase of the treatment. Once the limb is decongested and the patient wears compression garments, moisturizers should be applied twice daily.

Moisturizers, soaps or other skin cleansers used in lymphedema management, should have good moisturizing qualities, contain no fragrances, don't cause allergic reactions, and should be in either the neutral or acidic range of the pH scale, which is around pH 5.

Skincare products should first be tested on healthy skin prior to the initial application to areas affected by lymphedema in order to avoid allergic reactions. Products often used by lymphedema patients include Eucerin, Aquaphor, Lymphoderm, Lindi Skin products, Curel, and Johnson&Johnson Baby Lotion.

Other sources for skin irritations may be compression sleeves or stockings that are too tight, and materials used in compression bandaging. In these cases switching to other materials may remedy the problem.

Insect repellents should be applied in regions where mosquitoes are prevalent. To take proper care of mosquito bites and minor injuries, it is advisable to always carry an alcohol swab, antibacterial ointment, and a band-aid.

Tattoos in areas affected by lymphedema should be avoided; there are serious possible side effects associated with these procedures, such as infections, allergic reactions to ink pigments and carriers used, MRI complications(13), and blood-borne diseases. In addition, new findings indicate that metal particles from tattoo needles have been found in lymph nodes(12).

When caring for nails, it is important to keep the risk of infections to a minimum. Finger and toenails should be kept short using clippers instead of scissors; toenails should be cut straight across, and a podiatrist should be consulted to treat and prevent ingrown toenails. Cuticles on fingers and toes should not be cut but pushed back.

Acrylic nails should be avoided; bacteria between natural and artificial nails are a common cause of infections.

3.2.2 Two-Phase Approach of Complete Decongestive Therapy

Complete Decongestive Therapy (CDT) is applied in two phases; phase one, also known as the intensive or decongestive phase, is administered daily by a trained and certified lymphedema therapist (CLT). The main goal in this phase is to mobilize stagnated lymphatic fluid and to soften and decrease proliferated connective tissue present in lymphedema. Other goals include patient education in individualized exercise techniques, skin care, self-management techniques, and the long-term management of lymphedema.

Phase 1: CDT components in this phase include manual lymph drainage (MLD), compression therapy with padded short-stretch bandages, skin care and decongestive exercises.

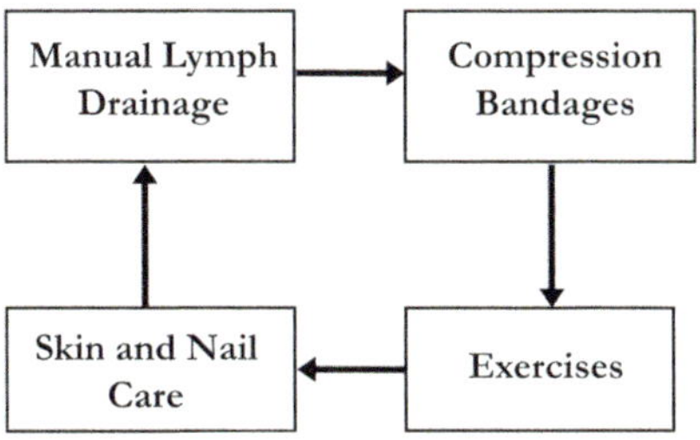

Fig. 3.16 CDT components in phase 1 of treatment

The overall goal is to re-route the lymph flow, including excess protein and water, around the blocked areas into more centrally located healthy lymph vessels and lymph nodes in order to decongest the affected body part to a normal or near normal size.

The severity and location of the lymphedematous swelling determines the duration of the intensive phase. In general, 2-3 weeks of daily treatments are necessary for individuals with lymphedema affecting the arm, and 2-4 weeks for lymphedema affecting the leg. In extreme cases, the decongestive phase may last up to 6 to 8 weeks and may have to be repeated several times in order to achieve satisfactory results.

Dosing for CDT in the intensive phase: Ideally, patients should be treated daily with a duration of 60-90 minutes at a time. The European model of CDT includes the administration of treatments twice a day until satisfactory results are achieved. This model is modified in the US to once daily treatment sessions 4-5 times per week.

In order for CDT to work most effectively, patients need to be treated daily. Changes in volume of the treated extremity can be drastic following treatments, and the application of short-stretch bandages applied following the MLD treatments preserves the decongestive results. The daily application of bandages is crucial to accommodate changes in volume and to prevent re-accumulation of evacuated lymph fluid. The bandages are worn by the patient between treatments, that is 23 hours per day. If treatments are limited to twice or three times per week, the bandages tend to slide and fluid starts to build up again in areas previously treated. In this scenario, therapists and patients are playing "catch-up" in each treatment session, and results are generally unsatisfactory. Bandages should not be removed by the patient at home. By removing the bandages in the treatment facility, the therapist will be able to determine if more padding is needed, or if the tension of compression bandages needs to be adjusted by inspecting the skin for pressure marks. Covering the bandages with cast covers, or a plastic bag, enables the patient to shower between treatments.

In the *Position Statement of the National Lymphedema Network for the Diagnosis and Treatment of Lymphedema*[(14)], it is stated that "Optimally, CDT should be performed daily (5 days/week) until the reduction of fluid volume has reached a plateau, which can take 3 to 8 weeks. Some patients may have good results from CDT with modifications of the frequency and duration of treatment. CDT frequency and duration should be individualized to produce the greatest reduction of swelling and improvement of skin condition in the shortest period of time."

The *International Lymphedema Framework's Best Practice for the Management of Lymphedema*[(15)] states that "Patients undergoing standard intensive therapy must be carefully selected and be willing and able to commit physically and emotionally to daily intensive therapy, including participation in exercise programs."

Both statements underline the necessity of daily lymphedema treatments, as well as patient motivation and compliance to achieve best results.

Compromises are sometimes necessary since every case of lymphedema is different, and there is no clear-cut approach to treatment. Treatment frequency and intensity depend on a multitude of factors, such as severity and stage of the swelling, the age and general physical condition of the patient, as well as existing comorbidities, such as congestive heart failure (CHF), diabetes, etc.

There are also healthcare-related limitations, such as out-of-pocket expenses (co-payments for treatments, cost for compression supplies), transportation issues, and general healthcare limits, which unfortunately seem to be the main reason for limitations and sub-optimal dosing for lymphedema treatment.

In a national survey labeled "*Lymphedema Therapists' Dosing of CDT in Breast Cancer Survivors with Lymphedema*"[(16)], published December 2017 in the Internet Journal of Allied Health Sciences and Practice (IJAHSP), it was reported that, in regard to the frequency, the average number of patient visits per week during Phase 1 of CDT was 3.71, according to the Physical Therapists, Occupational Therapists, Physical Therapist Assistants and Occupational Therapists Assistants trained in lymphedema therapy, that participated in that survey.

This number is clearly below the recommended weekly dosage for CDT in Phase 1. One of the main reasons for not following the daily recommended dosing of CDT listed in the IJAHSP survey was that "*the therapists' dosage determination was impacted by their perception of the patients' readiness and adherence to lymphedema treatment and self-management.*"

Patient motivation and compliance are imperative to achieving optimal treatment results; it is, therefore, necessary to explain the treatment protocol and recommended dosage to the patient. Patients need to be aware that less than five treatment sessions per week during the first two weeks in the intensive phase will lead to an increased number of treatment sessions and a longer overall treatment time. Most informed patients recognize that trading fewer weekly visits in exchange for an increased overall treatment time with most likely poorer results, is an unfavorable deal.

CDT is most effective if performed five times per week for a minimum of two weeks in most patients. After that, treatment dosage may be reduced to three times per week, if necessary, until the lymphedema is decongested, and the patient can be measured for a compression garment. The most substantial reduction in lymphedema volume generally occurs within the first week of treatment.

Patients should be treated Monday through Friday and instructed to wear the bandages over the treatment-free weekend. Adherence to this recommended dosage will yield better treatment outcomes and less overall treatment visits. If treatments are applied only 2 to 3 times a week, the patient may be without treatment for 3 or 4 days that week; in that case, patients and therapists are fighting an uphill battle caused by sliding bandages in days without treatment and subsequent re-accumulation of fluid in the affected extremity. This will inevitably lead to poor treatment outcomes, an increased overall length of treatment time and patient visits, as well as frustration on both the therapists' and the patients' sides.

Phase 2: The end of the first phase of CDT is determined by the results of measurements on the affected body part, which are taken by the therapist. Once measurements approach a flat line, the end of phase one is reached, and the patient progresses seamlessly into phase two of CDT, also known as the self-management phase. CDT components in this phase include self-MLD, compression therapy with compression garments, skin care and individualized exercises.

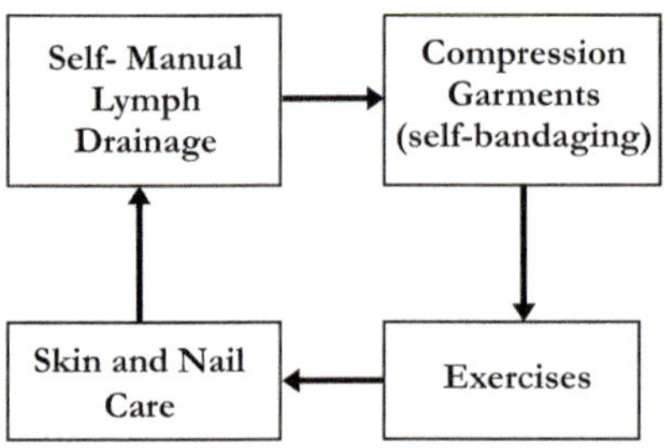

Fig. 3.17 CDT components in phase 2 of treatment

Phase two is an ongoing and individualized part of CDT, in which the patient assumes responsibility for maintaining and improving the treatment results achieved in the first phase of CDT.

During the intensive phase, the patients are instructed in the individual components of self-management, which include a skin care regimen, home exercises, self-manual lymph drainage and the application of compression garments for daytime use. In some cases, it may be necessary for the patient to apply padded compression bandages, or alternative compression devices for night-time use. Regular check-ups with the physician and the lymphedema therapist during phase two are necessary.

For more information on self-management techniques, see 3.6.Self-Management of Lymphedema.

3.3 Pneumatic Compression

A pneumatic compression device (PCD) for the treatment of lymphedema consists of an electrical pneumatic pump and an inflatable garment with multiple pressure compartments that is applied on the extremity; most manufacturers offer garment extensions that cover the adjacent trunkal quadrants. The air pump inflates the garment intermittently with compressed air and deflates with cycle times and pressures that vary between devices.

Inflatable garments in older generation PCDs only offer single pressure compartments, whereas newer generation devices have multiple compartments and air pumps that are equipped with programmable options and calibrated pressure. The compartments in newer generation pumps inflate sequentially from the lower part to the upper part of the extremity until all segments are fully inflated, thereby creating a pressure gradient, which is important to effectively move stagnated fluid. Following this phase, all compartments deflate at the same time. PCDs labeled as Type III pumps are advanced segmented devices with calibrated gradient pressure and are further characterized by a manual control on at least three outflow ports of the device that can deliver an individually determined pressure to each compartment of the unit. It is possible to make manual adjustments in the pressure in the individual compartments and/or the length and frequency of the inflation cycles.

Fig 3.18 Flexitouch® Plus Advanced Pneumatic Compression Device (a) lower extremity; (b) upper extremity application. With permission from Tactile Medical

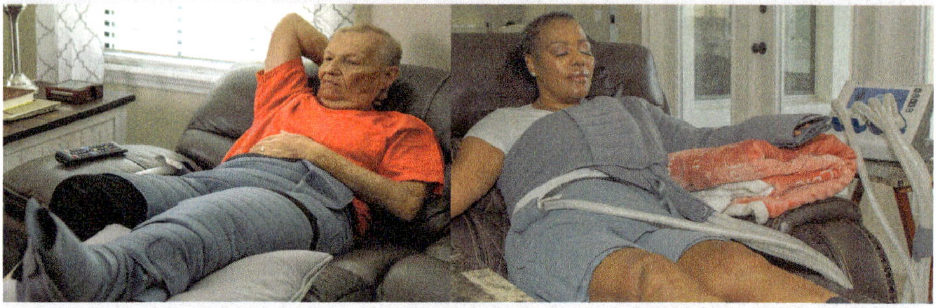

(a) (b)

Consensus on the proper pressure level and treatment duration in PCDs for the treatment of lymphedema is lacking. Generally, the pressure level should be adjusted to the patient's degree of tolerance and response to treatment. Careful instruction of the patient in the use of these devices and surveillance by a practitioner trained on a specialist level in these devices is required.

A review of the literature suggests that recommendations for pressure levels are inconsistent, ranging between 5 to over 120 mm/Hg[19]; study data indicates that sustained high pressures over a long period of time can cause skin damage as a result of diminished blood supply, and that sustained pressure settings of 60-70 mm/Hg should be considered the upper limit. Peak inflation pressure of 25-60 mmHg may be sufficient for treatment settings in most patients[15,18]. A treatment duration of 30 minutes to two hours, one hour twice a day, is generally recommended. Careful guidance by a practitioner with knowledge in lymphedema treatment is mandatory to determine optimal treatment frequency.

The use of PCDs in the treatment of lymphedema is neither accepted as a replacement, nor a part of complete decongestive therapy; pneumatic compression cannot replace CDT as the recognized gold standard for the treatment of lymphedema and should not be used as a stand-alone therapy for lymphedema. However, recent studies suggest that there is a potential place for newer generation Type III PCD devices as an adjunct treatment modality to control lymphedema, especially for patients with limited access to medical care, or if physical limitations of the individual may result in challenges controlling the lymphedema independently in the self-administered phase 2 of CDT.

PCDs are proven to be effective in removing water from the tissues; however, evidence suggests that proteins remain in the affected areas in lymphedema[18] following the use of PCDs. This may have long-term negative effects on lymphedema and calls into question if the volume reduction with the use of pneumatic compression for lymphedema management can be sustained over longer periods of time.

The Centers for Medicare and Medicaid Services (CMS) cover pneumatic compression devices in the home setting for the treatment of lymphedema only if the patient has undergone a four-week trial of conservative therapy (CDT) and the treating physician determines that there has been no significant improvement or if significant symptoms remain after the trial[17].

It is important to point out that compression therapy with bandages and/ or garments must be continued following the use of pneumatic compression devices to prevent a rebound of swelling.

Optimal treatment and management of lymphedema always necessitate a treatment approach that is tailored to the patient's specific needs; PCDs devices can be an additional tool in a multi-modality approach to effectively treat lymphedema.

The following contraindications are listed in the Lymphedema Framework's international consensus document "*Best Practice Guideline for Lymphedema*"[15]:

- Non-pitting chronic lymphedema
- Known or suspected deep vein thrombosis
- Pulmonary embolism
- Thrombophlebitis
- Acute inflammation of the skin (erysipelas, cellulitis)

- Uncontrolled/severe cardiac failure
- Pulmonary edema
- Ischemic vascular disease
- Active metastatic diseases affecting the edematous region
- Edema at the root of the extremity or trunkal edema
- Severe peripheral neuropathy

3.4 Surgical Treatment

Various surgical procedures for the treatment of lymphedema have been practiced for over a century, and advancements in medical technologies have led to increased discussion of the role of surgical treatment as a supplementary option for a select group of lymphedema patients.

While research shows that surgical management of lymphedema has beneficial effects for some patients, there is a broad consensus that conservative, non-surgical management of lymphedema remains the first line of standard care, and that surgical procedures do not eliminate the need for complete decongestive therapy prior to and following surgical procedures(14,20,21), and should act only as a supplement to conservative treatment options.

Surgical modalities should be reserved for patients who did not achieve satisfactory results with conservative treatments, or when the achieved success of conservative protocols can no longer be maintained(3). Surgery may also be considered when the excess weight of the affected extremity is a main contributing factor to functional impairment and cosmetic deformity, and to reduce the frequency of inflammations.

The potential benefit of any surgical procedure should be compared to the risks associated with it. The medical expertise in lymphedema of the surgical team, as well as good cooperation between the surgeons and lymphedema therapist should also be a major point of consideration(14), since conservative treatments are still necessary following surgical care.

In general, surgical approaches can be classified as excisional techniques, reconstructive techniques, and tissue transfer procedures.

3.4.1 Liposuction

Other terms to describe this excisional surgical technique include Suction Assisted Lipectomy (SAL), Circumferential Suction Assisted Lipectomy (CSAL), and Suction Assisted Protein Lipectomy (SAPL).

Liposuction is the most common procedure in cosmetic surgery; however, the surgical techniques used in lymphedema surgery are very different than cosmetic liposuction and should not be performed by surgeons unfamiliar with lymphedema and without significant training and experience with these techniques.

Modern suction-assisted surgical lipectomy is a procedure that can effectively remove the excess fibrotic and fatty tissues that have permanently accumulated in chronic lymphedema and cannot be removed with conservative treatment modalities. This procedure must be offered as part of a comprehensive treatment system that includes conservative lymphedema therapy (CDT), which is administered prior to the surgical procedure to address excess fluid components present in lymphedema. The volume reduction achieved with liposuction modalities are permanent with the ongoing use of custom-fitting compression garments following the surgery.

Liposuction removes excess deposits of solids and fatty tissue but does not address the pathophysiological processes that lead to the accumulation of fluids in lymphedema. Therefore, lymphedema can still recur following liposuction, and patients who underwent this procedure have to continue lifelong wearing of custom-fitted compression garments. The integration of individualized lymphedema therapy and compression garment use following liposuction surgery is critical in achieving and maintaining good results. An average volume reduction of 111% in arms and 86% in legs have been reported following surgery [(24)]. Patients who are unable to maintain long-term compression post-liposuction are not good candidates for this surgery.

The literature suggests that liposuction surgery has proven to be safe if performed by experienced and knowledgeable surgeons and that additional impairment to the lymphatic transport was not associated with this surgical modality[(23)].

3.4.2 Reconstructive Surgical Techniques

Lymphatic reconstructive procedures attempt to improve the rate of lymphatic return to the blood circulation. Techniques include transplant of functioning lymph vessels, lymph nodes, or veins from other areas of the body from the same individual (autologous), into those areas affected by lymphedema, and the direct connection of these lymph vessels and nodes to neighboring veins.

These procedures are mostly used in the earlier stages of lymphedema (before the occurrence of fibrotic and adipose tissues), in which the fluid component is predominantly responsible for the excess volume. Recent advances in micro-surgical procedures and instruments used, as well as improved imaging techniques led to continued progress in these procedures, and reductions in limb volume have been reported.

Lympho-Lymphatic Anastomosis (LLA):

This procedure involves the autologous harvesting of healthy, functioning lymph vessels and transferring these vessels to the area affected by lymphedema, where they are sutured directly to the lymph vessels in the limb affected by lymphedema. The goal is to improve or restore lymphatic flow by creating a bridge bypassing the scarred or radiated area. The healthy lymph vessels used in this procedure are usually taken from the inner thigh region; there is a theoretical risk of inducing lymphedema at the donor site.

Lympho-Venous Anastomosis (LVA):

This procedure relies on the artificial connection of lymphatic vessels in the area affected by lymphedema to small adjacent superficial veins (venules), allowing lymph fluid to directly drain into the venous system, thus bypassing areas of obstructed lymph flow. Better results tend to be achieved in early stage lymphedema and when numerous lymphatic-venous anastomoses are performed; upper extremity lymphedema tends to show better results than lymphedema affecting the legs[25]. No donor site is required for this procedure, which makes this procedure the least invasive with the lowest surgical risk.

Vacularized Lymph Node Transfer (VLNT):

In this procedure soft tissue containing lymph nodes with their arterial and venous blood vessels from the same individual (autologous) is harvested from a donor site (groin, chest wall, or neck) and transplanted to the area affected by lymphedema. Here, the blood vessels of the donor tissue are connected to local blood vessels to re-establish the blood supply to the transferred nodes. New lymphatic vessels are expected to sprout from the transplanted nodes and remaining lymph vessels are expected to re-grow, thus restoring lymphatic drainage and preventing the formation of new scar tissue.

While reported outcomes of VLNT in literature have been promising[25], it should be noted that all surgical procedures are invasive, costly, involve significant risks, and the long-term results are not yet known. Conservative management of lymphedema with complete decongestive therapy is noninvasive, with minimal to no side effects for patients, shows excellent long-term results, and should always be the primary treatment of choice.

3.5 Pharmaceuticals

Diuretics

These drugs promote salts and fluid in the body to be excreted. Although diuretics may be beneficial in the short-term and may be indicated in those cases when lymphedema is associated with other conditions, such as congestive heart failure, renal and liver disease, or hypertension, they may be harmful and contribute to the worsening of lymphedema related symptoms if used long-term. There is no evidence that diuretics improve the function of the lymphatic system[15].

Diuretics used for lymphedema are limited to removing the water content of the swelling, while the protein molecules remain in the soft tissues. The dehydration effect of diuretics causes a higher concentration of the protein mass in the edema fluid, which may cause the tissues to become more fibrotic and increase the potential for secondary inflammations. In addition, the remaining proteins characteristically draw more water to the swollen areas as soon as the diuretic loses its effectiveness and may cause the volume of the lymphedema to increase.

The *2020 Consensus Document of the International Society of Lymphology* states: "Diuretic agents are occasionally useful during the initial treatment phase of complete decongestive therapy (CDT). Long-term administration, however, is discouraged for its marginal benefits in the treatment of peripheral lymphedema and potentially may induce fluid and electrolyte imbalance"[(3)].

Benzopyrones

These drugs include Coumarin and bioflavonoids and have been shown to promote the breakdown of proteins present in lymphedema. Research has shown that their practical usefulness in the treatment of lymphedema is questionable. The United States and Australia abandoned the use of Coumarin due to liver toxicity and lack of effectiveness[(21,26)].

Antibiotics

Individuals who are at high risk for lymphedema must remain alert to the signs of infection as these symptoms are often the first indication for the onset of lymphedema. In such cases, quick intervention may help to delay the onset of lymphedema, as well as prevent the infection. The problem may aggravate and become potentially life-threatening if timely care is not taken.

Antibiotics should be administered as soon as possible; penicillin based medications are used either orally if no systemic infection is present, or by intravenous application. Oral penicillin is administered for a minimum of 14 days, or until the inflammation has been resolved. In some patients, it may take one or two months of therapy for symptoms to completely resolve. Other antibiotics may be used in cases of penicillin allergy (clindamycin or clarithromycin). In severe cases, hospitalization may be necessary. Prophylactic antibiotic therapy may be used in some instances to prevent recurrent infections in patients with lymphedema[27]. Newer research indicates that non-steroidal anti-inflammatory drugs (NSAID), such as Ketoprofen may be able to reduce recurrent infections and ease other symptoms associated with lymphedema[28].

Antimicrobials

Fungal infections in patients with lymphedema are common and should be treated with antimycotic pharmaceuticals. It is recommended to wash the affected area with a mild disinfectant, the anti-fungal drug is then applied to the dry skin according to the manufacturers recommendation[3].

3.6 Self-Management

To maintain the treatment success achieved in the intensive phase of CDT (see 3.2.2) and to further improve the volume reduction of the affected extremity and soften areas of increased and hardened tissues, patients are instructed in home-care and self-management techniques consisting of self-bandaging and self-manual lymph drainage (self-MLD), skin care and exercise modalities by the lymphedema therapist during phase 1 of therapy.

3.6.1 Self-Manual Lymph Drainage

The main objective in self-MLD is to re-route the lymph fluid around damaged or blocked areas, and to move the fluid towards healthy lymph vessels and nodes. From there, the lymph fluid returns to the venous system in the area of the venous angles, which are located on the base of the neck, just above and behind the collar bone. (Fig. 1.3). Every self-MLD sequence begins with stationary circles on the base of the neck, and after that the healthy drainage areas are manipulated in order to stimulate the lymph vessels and nodes that are responsible to move the fluid from the area affected by lymphedema. This sequence application improves the activity of these lymph vessels, thereby creating a "suction effect" on the area where the lymph fluid is trapped. Only when these drainage areas are properly prepared, the self-MLD sequence will include the lymphatic pathways on the affected extremity from the top to the bottom. The treatment sequences are customized for upper and lower extremity lymphedema and vary dependent on which side is affected. For example, if the right arm is affected, the sequence will be 1. the neck, 2. the lymph nodes in the left axilla, 3. the lymphatic pathways from the right to the left axilla, 4. the lymph nodes in the right groin, 5. the lymphatic pathways from the right axilla to the right groin, and finally 6. from the right shoulder down to the fingers of the right arm.

Important Aspects in Self-MLD:

- Don't start self-MLD without proper instruction by your lymphedema therapist. The main stroke used in self-MLD is the stationary circle (see 3.2.1); you need to be familiar with the technique, the pressure and the particular treatment sequence for your condition.
- Pressure: having completed the intensive phase with your certified therapist, you should be familiar with the gentle pressure used in MLD, which should be just enough to stretch the skin to it's maximum elasticity, but not enough to feel the muscles, or tendons beneath the skin. The amount of pressure is often compared to the pressure applied stroking a newborns head, or when pressure is applied to the eyelid, no discomfort should be felt on the eyeball.
- Working and resting pressure: the common denominator of all strokes, including stationary circles, is the resting and working phase. Imagining a circle, the working phase would be the first half of the circle, in which the pressure gradually increases and decreases in the direction you want the lymph fluid to move. In the working phase of the stroke, lymphatic structures located in the fatty tissues of the skin are gently stretched, resulting in an increase in their activity. Once the first half circle is completed, the hand relaxes completely, but maintains contact with the skin. In this resting phase, the elasticity of the skin carries the hand back to the starting position without any applied pressure; then the circle is repeated. Use the skin's elasticity and do not slide over the skin while performing stationary circles; use as much hand surface as possible, not just the finger tips, in order to maximize the surface area of each stroke.

- Ideally, each stroke should be repeated 10-15 times within a sequence; the entire self-MLD treatment should last between 10 and 15 minutes and be performed at least once per day, more if needed. Self-MLD should be followed by the application of skin moisturizers and compression therapy.
- If the MLD sequence for your condition includes pressure applied to the deep abdominal area, you should consult with your therapist for any possible contraindications, such as recent surgery or radiation to the abdominal area, diverticulitis, Crohn's disease, pregnancy, others.
- Any kind of skin irritation needs to be addressed promptly, specifically if cellulitis is suspected, in which case self-treatment has to be suspended until antibiotics are taken and the symptoms have improved.
- Make sure you are in a comfortable position while performing self-MLD to avoid straining other areas of your body, such as the back or neck.
- Finally, learning self-MLD techniques is essential to taking control of your lymphedema. Should you be unsure of any hand placement or pressure direction, please consult with your lymphedema therapist.

The following sequences for upper and lower extremity lymphedema include basic and easy to follow techniques, and do not include all sequences and techniques used by your lymphedema therapist.

The sequences may have to be adjusted to your individual situation, including any physical limitations being present. You can review these techniques with your lymphedema therapist, who will modify and/or exclude/add certain techniques if necessary.

Upper Extremity Lymphedema Sequence

The hand techniques used for this sequence are stationary circles and effleurage, which is a gentle stroking motion applied with the flat hand sliding over the skin. Effleurage is the only MLD stroke that allows sliding, all other strokes are applied using skin elasticity without sliding.

1. Stationary circles on the base of the neck behind the collar bone on both sides. Place as many fingers as possible flatly to the area; the working phase of the circle is directed outward and forward, staying behind the collar bone. Manipulate each side separately (switching hands), or simultaneously (right hand left side, and vice versa) (Fig. 3.19).

2. Stationary circles in the center of the opposite underarm (axillary lymph nodes). The flat hand is placed in a longitudinal plane with the pressure in the working half of the circle directed to the back and center of the axilla (Fig. 3.20). If your left arm is affected, manipulate the right side; the left axilla is treated with lymphedema on the right arm.

3. Apply an effleurage from the affected axillary area to the other side using the flat hand, fingers and palm, with gentle pressure (Fig. 3.21).

4. Stationary circles from the affected axillary area to the other side using the flat hand. Pressure is directed upward and to the other side in several placements until the entire area between the axillary regions is covered (Fig. 3.22).

5. Stationary circles in the groin on the affected side (right groin with arm lymphedema on the right, left groin with lymphedema on the left arm). The goal is to manipulate the inguinal lymph nodes located in the groin with the flat hand positioned below the inguinal ligament on the top of your thigh. Pressure is applied to the middle of the thigh and towards the belly (Fig. 3.23).

6. Stationary circles from the affected axillary area toward the groin on the same side using the flat hand on the side of your body in a direct line between the axilla and groin. Pressure is directed toward the back and downward in several placements until the entire area between the axillary region and the groin is covered (Fig. 3.24).

7. Stationary circles on top of the shoulder on the side where your lymphedema is located. Pressure with the entire flat hand positioned in a horizontal plane is directed toward the back and the neck in several placements until the entire upper shoulder area is covered (Fig. 3.25).

8. Apply an effleurage using the flat hand, fingers and palm, with gentle

pressure covering the entire arm from the fingers to the shoulder (Fig. 3.26).

9. Apply stationary circles on the side of your affected arm with the flat hand in several placements from the shoulder down to the elbow. The pressure is directed toward the back and upward in the direction of the shoulder. The pressure should not be directed toward the axillary area, but to the shoulder (Fig. 3.27).

10. Apply stationary circles from the inside of the upper arm toward the side of the upper arm. The pressure is directed toward the side of the upper arm and to the shoulder area. Use several hand placements until the entire upper arm area is covered. The pressure should not be directed toward the axillary area, but to the shoulder (Fig. 3.28).

11. Stationary circles are applied to the remaining arm, including the front of the elbow, the front and back of the forearm, hand and fingers. Pressure is directed toward the side of the arm and in the direction of the shoulder area in all placements until the entire elbow, forearm and hand are covered. (Figs. 3.29-3.32).

12. Re-work the following areas in reverse once you are finished: Steps #9 to #1.

Following this treatment sequence, appropriate skin moisturizers should be applied, and the compression garment or compression bandages should be placed on the arm. Exercises are ideally performed following self-MLD with the compression garment or bandages in place.

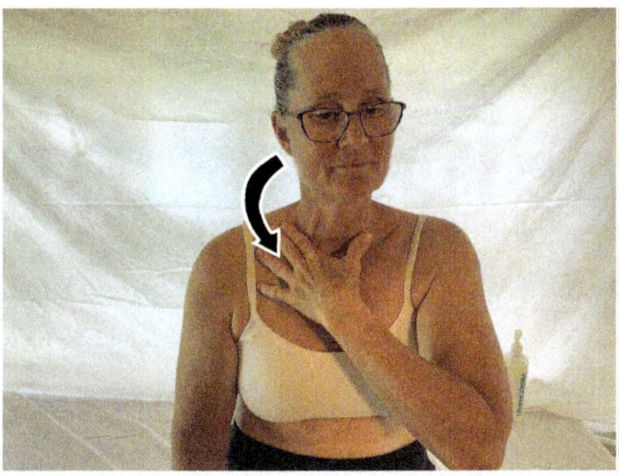

Fig. 3.19

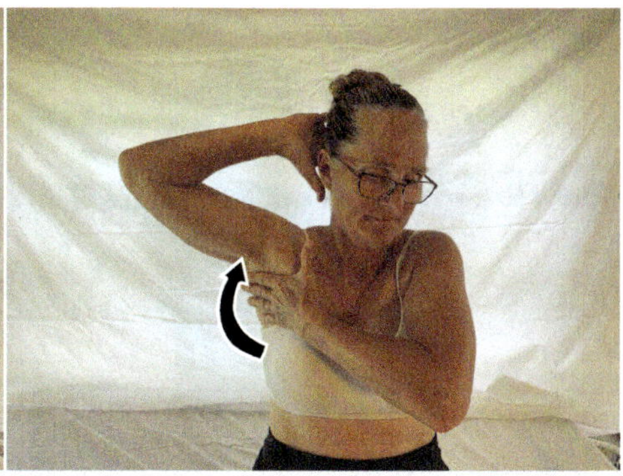

Fig. 3.20

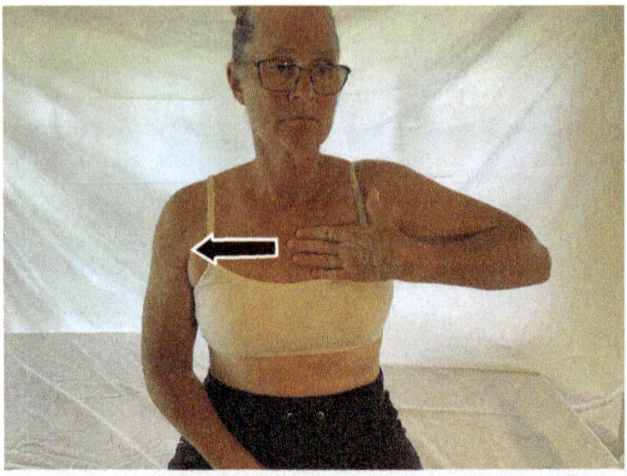

Fig. 3.21

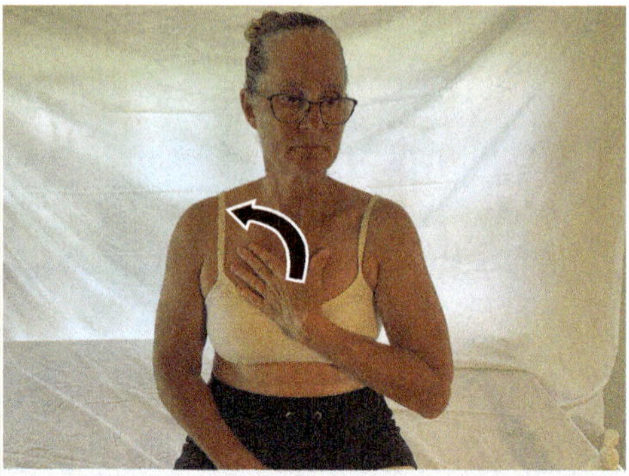

Fig. 3.22

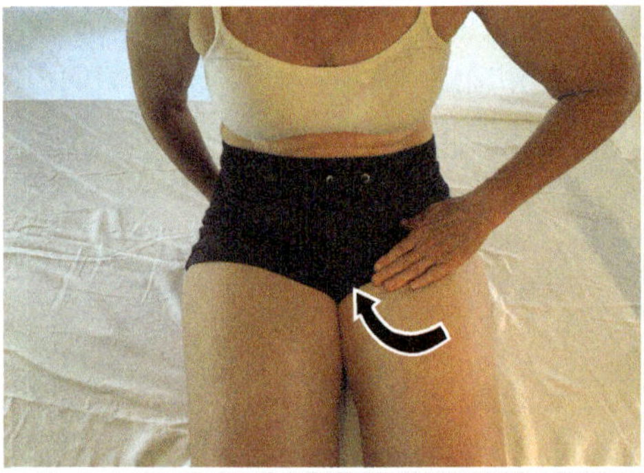

Fig. 3.23

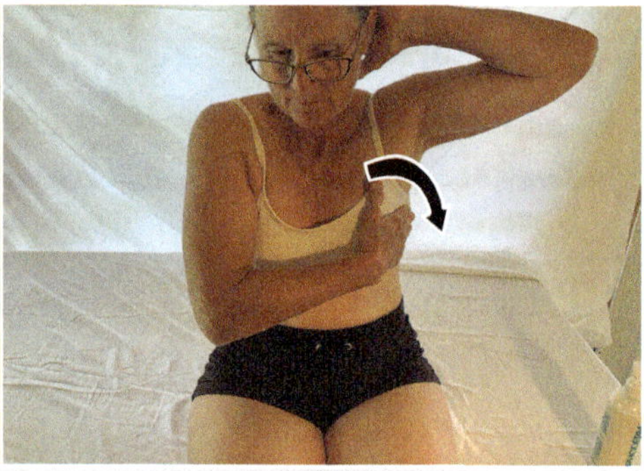

Fig. 3.24

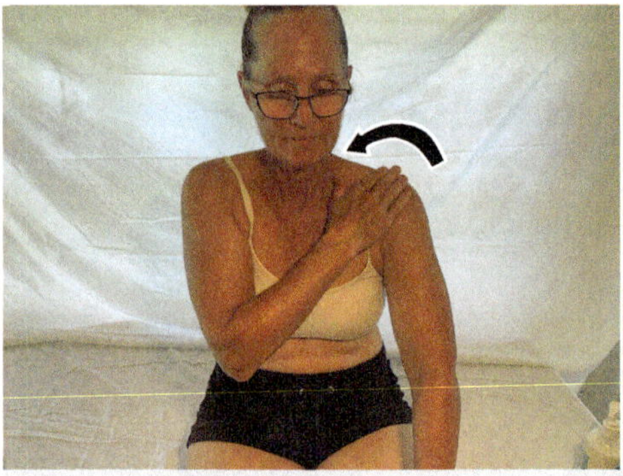

Fig. 3.25

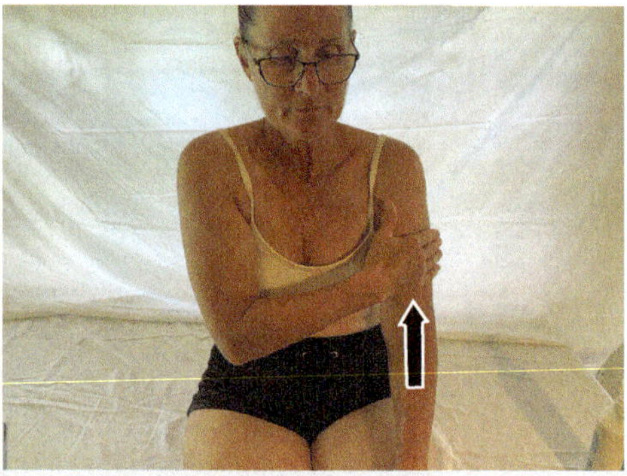

Fig. 3.26

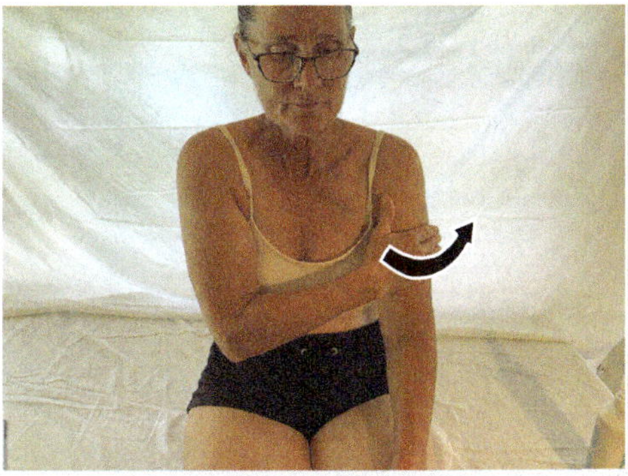

Fig. 3.27

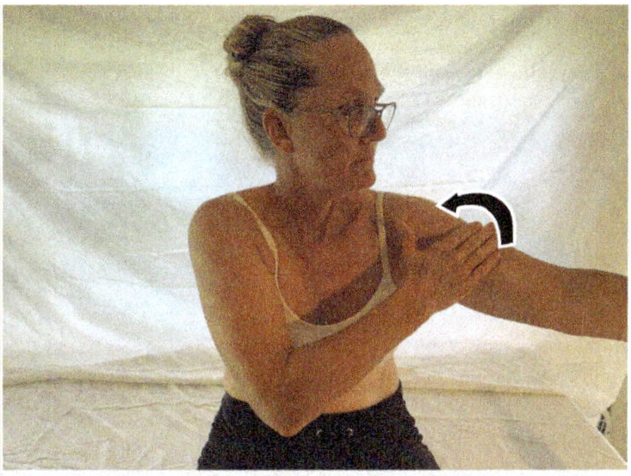

Fig. 3.28

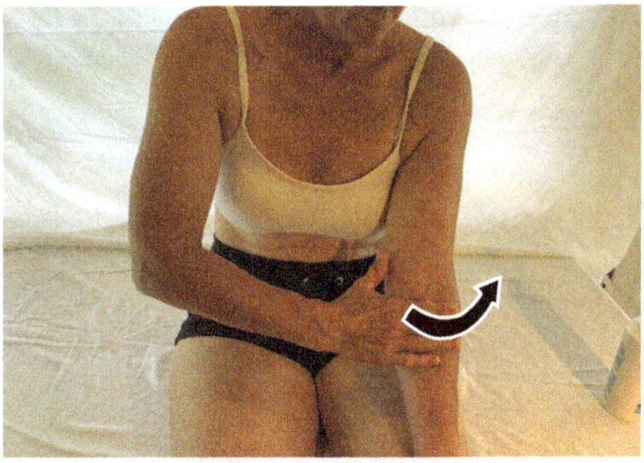

Fig. 3.29

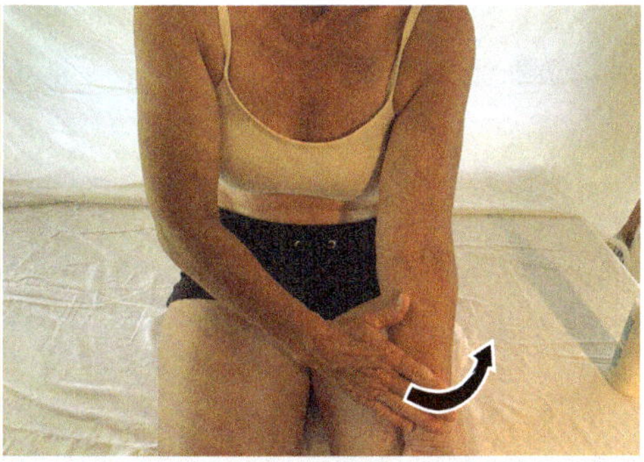

Fig. 3.30

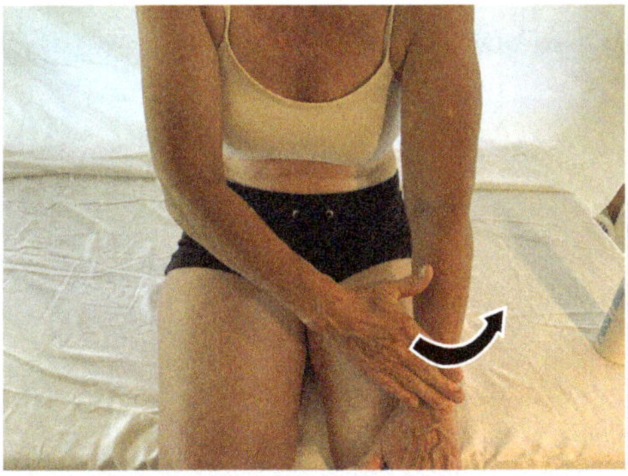

Fig. 3.31

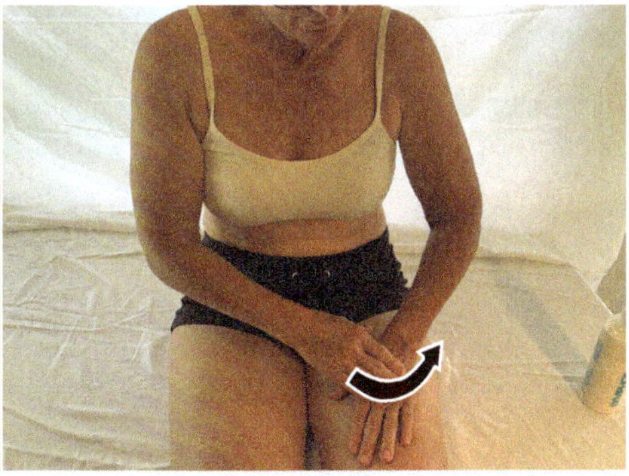

Fig. 3.32

Abdominal breathing exercises may be performed following the treatment sequence for the arm to maximize lymph flow.

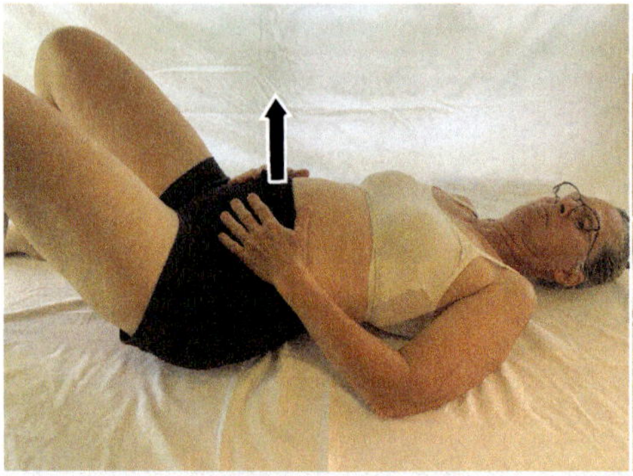

Fig. 3.33

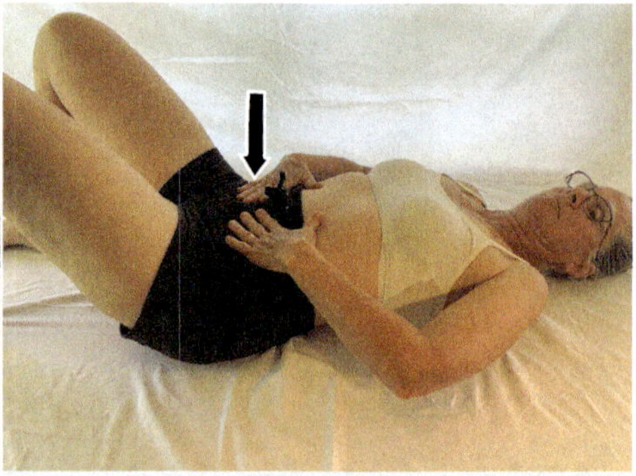

Fig. 3.34

To perform these exercises place both hands flat on your belly lying in a supine position with your knees bent and a small pillow under your head; these diaphragmatic breathing exercises can also be performed sitting comfortably on a chair.

Inhale through your nose against your hands into the belly, so that you feel your stomach rising against your flat hands. Exhale slowly with your lips pursed and your hands gently following the belly down to your spine and slightly upward into the chest. Repeat 5-10 times. Should you feel dizzy, or if the downward movement causes discomfort, stop. Prior to performing deep breathing exercises consult with your therapist for any possible contraindications, such as recent surgery or radiation to the abdominal area, diverticulitis, and others (Figs. 3.33, 3.34).

Lower Extremity Lymphedema Sequence

The hand techniques used for this sequence are stationary circles and effleurage, which is a gentle stroking motion applied with the flat hand while sliding over the skin. Effleurage is the only MLD stroke that allows sliding; all other strokes are applied using skin elasticity without sliding. This sequence is ideally performed lying supine with knees slightly bent and a small pillow under your head. If the supine position is not possible, the sequence can also be performed sitting comfortable on a chair with the leg supported on a stool, or similar.

1. Stationary circles on the base of the neck behind the collar bone on both sides. Place as many fingers as possible flatly to the area; the working phase of the circle is directed outward and forward, staying behind the collar bone. Manipulate each side separately (switching hands), or simultaneously (right hand left side; vice versa) (Fig. 3.35).

2. Stationary circles in the center of the underarm (axillary lymph nodes) on the same side your lymphedema is located; If your left leg is affected, manipulate the left side; the right axilla is manipulated with lymphedema on the right leg. The flat hand is placed in a longitudinal plane with the pressure in the working half of the circle directed to the back and center of the axilla (Fig. 3.36).

3. Stationary circles with the flat hand (palm and fingers) from the waist of the side where the lymphedema is located to the axillary area on the same side, in a direct line between the waist and the underarm area. Pressure is directed toward the back and up in the direction of the axilla. Use several placements until the entire area between the waist and the underarm area on the same side is covered (Fig. 3.37).

4. Stationary circles in the groin on the unaffected side (right groin with leg lymphedema on the left, left groin with lymphedema on the right leg). The goal is to manipulate the inguinal lymph nodes located in the groin with the flat hand positioned below the inguinal ligament on top of your thigh. Pressure is applied to the middle of the thigh and towards the belly (Fig. 3.38).

5. Stationary circles from the affected groin (inguinal) area toward the groin on the other side using the flat hand positioned over the pubic area in a direct line between both groin areas. Pressure is directed downward and toward the groin of the unaffected side. Use several placements until the entire area between both sides is covered (Figs. 3.39, 3.40). One hand or both hands may be used simultaneously or alternating.

6. Abdominal (diaphragmatic) breathing exercises: Inhale through your nose

against your hands into the belly, so that you feel your stomach rising against your flat hands. Exhale slowly with your lips pursed and your hands gently following the belly down to your spine and slightly upward into the chest. Repeat 5-10 times. Should you feel dizzy, or if the downward movement causes discomfort, stop. Prior to performing deep breathing exercises consult with your therapist for any possible contraindications, such as recent surgery or radiation to the abdominal area, diverticulitis, and others (Figs. 3.41, 3.42). Sequences on the affected leg:

7. Apply an effleurage with flat hands covering the entire leg from the ankles all the way up toward the side of the thigh (Fig. 3.43).

8. Stationary circles with one or both hands on the side of your affected thigh. Use flat hand(s) in several placements from the knee up to the hip. The pressure is directed toward the back and upward in the direction of the hip. The pressure should not be directed toward the groin area, but to the hip/waist (Fig. 3.44).

9. Apply stationary circles with one or both hands from the inside toward the outside of the thigh. The pressure is directed toward the side of the thigh and to the hip area. Use several hand placements until the entire thigh area is covered. The pressure should not be directed toward the groin area, but to the hip/waist (Fig. 3.45).

10. Use stationary circles with the flat fingers of both hands behind the knee. The pressure is directed toward the thigh (Fig. 3.46).

11. Apply stationary circles with one or both hands on the inside of the knee and the lower leg in several placements between the knee and the inside ankle. The pressure is directed toward the thigh (Fig. 3.47).

12. Use stationary circles with the flat hands positioned on the inside and outside of the lower leg. The pressure is directed toward back and the thigh. Use several hand placements until the entire lower leg is covered (Fig. 3.48). Cover the back of the foot with stationary circles applied with one hand with the pressure directed toward the lower leg.

13. Re-work the entire leg in reverse with sequences #11 to #7. Then continue re-working the drainage areas with sequences #5 to #1, and finish the sequence with abdominal breathing described in sequence #6

Following this treatment sequence, appropriate skin moisturizers should be applied, and the compression garment or compression bandages should be placed to the leg. Exercises are ideally performed following self-MLD with the compression garment or bandages in place.

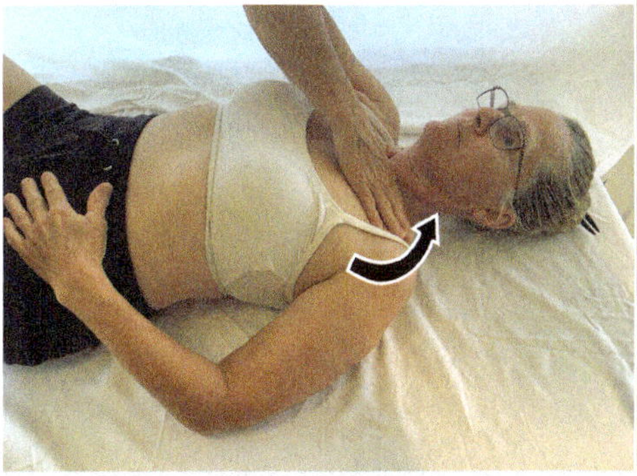
Fig. 3.35

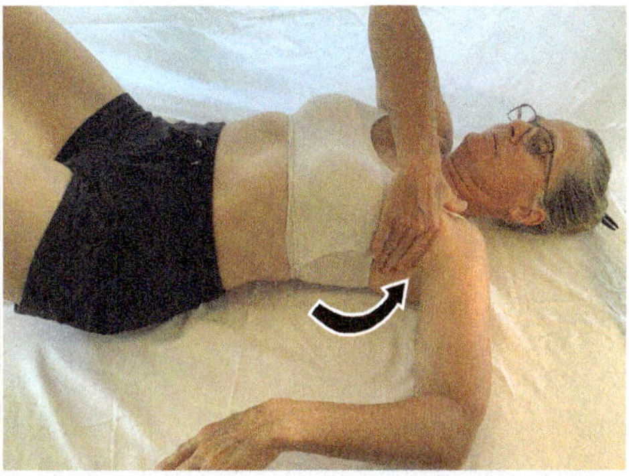
Fig. 3.36

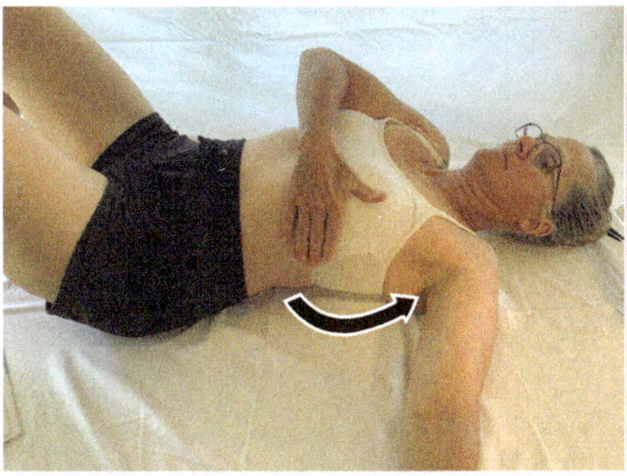
Fig. 3.37

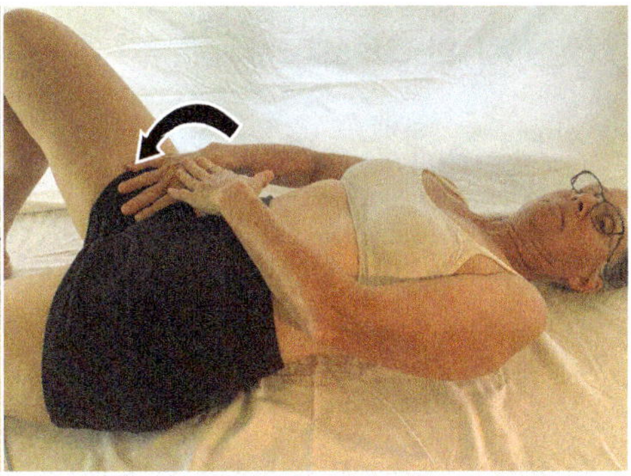
Fig. 3.38

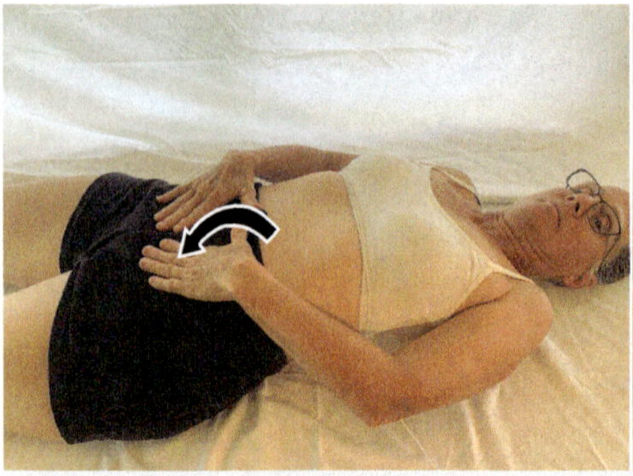

Fig. 3.39

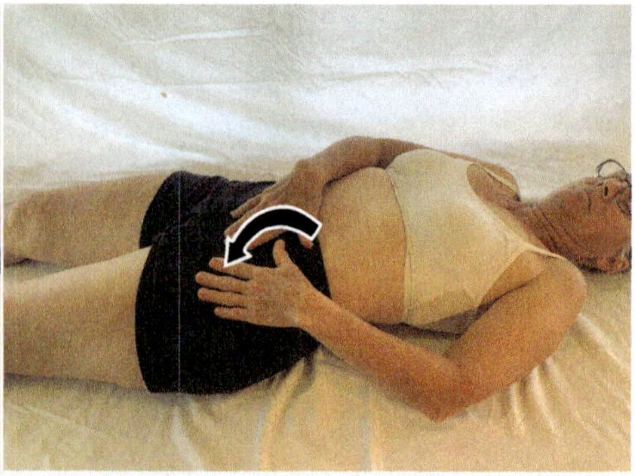

Fig. 3.40

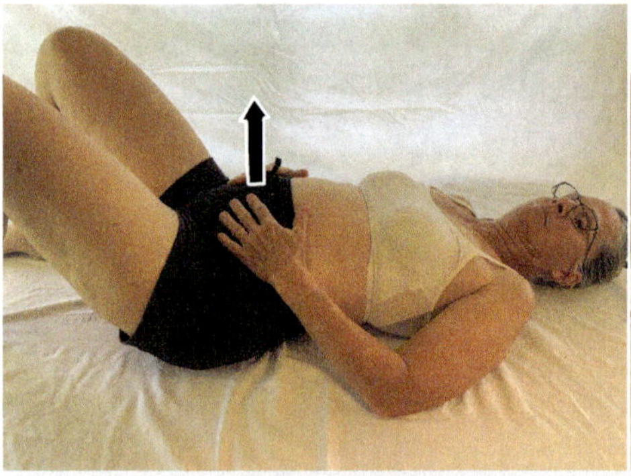

Fig. 3.41

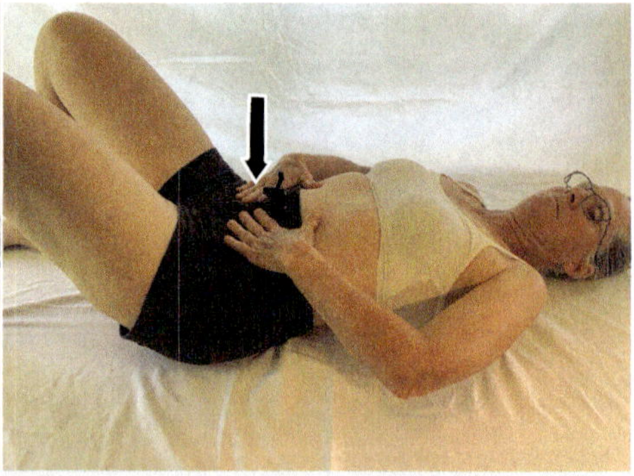

Fig. 3.42

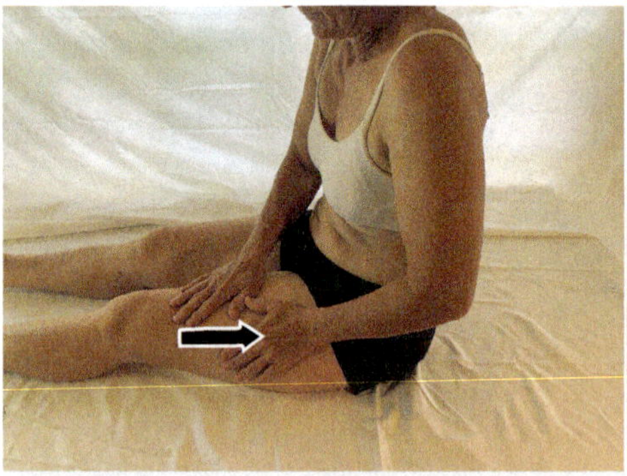

Fig. 3.43

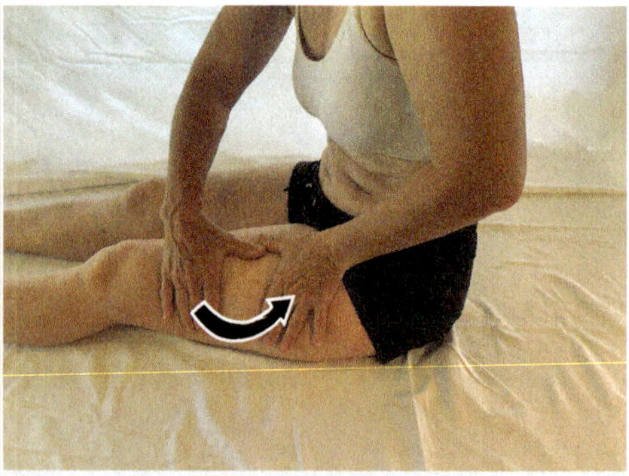

Fig. 3.44

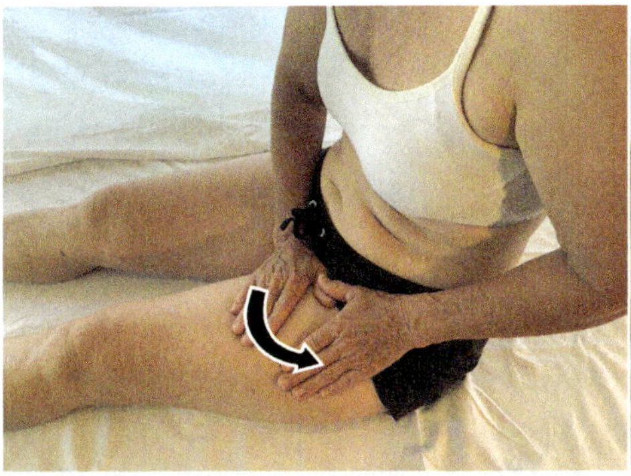

Fig. 3.45

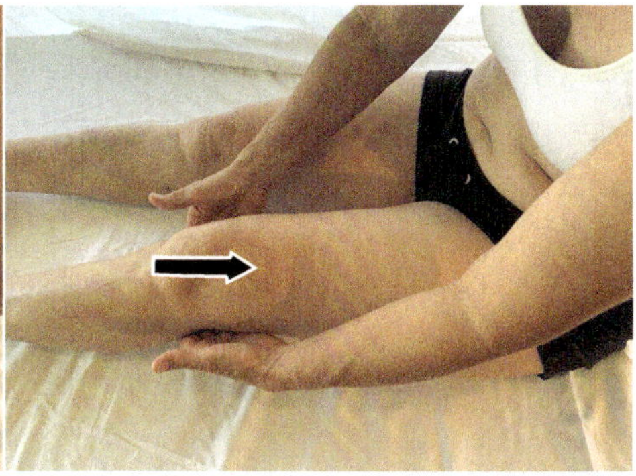

Fig. 3.46

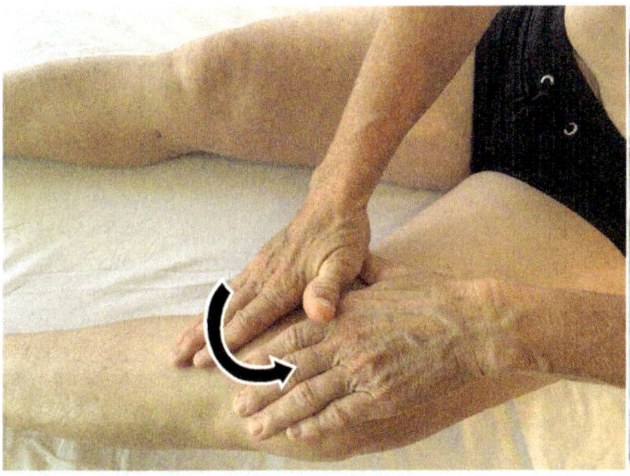

Fig. 3.47

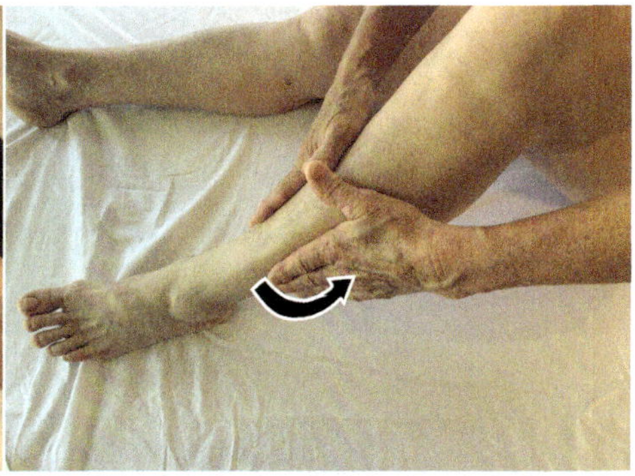

Fig. 3.48

3.6.2 Self-Bandaging

During the intensive phase of treatment, patients are instructed by the therapist to apply a simplified version of padded short-stretch compression bandages to the affected extremity. Having a good understanding in the application of bandages can be important in the intensive part of the treatment, also known as phase 1 of CDT, especially if bandages begin to slide over the treatment free weekend in this phase. Sliding is usually limited to the upper portion of the extremity; when it occurs, the bandages tend to bunch up, which may cause a tourniquet effect on the extremity and fluid to accumulate in these areas. Patients should be able to re-apply the compression bandages without difficulty in order to prevent these unwanted effects.

Knowing how to apply self-bandaging is also important in the second phase of CDT, in cases when lymphedema volume notably fluctuates throughout the day while the compression garment is worn. In order to counter this effect, it may be necessary to apply bandages at night whenever needed to maintain and improve the treatment results.

It is important to understand that self-bandaging must not be applied without proper instruction by the certified lymphedema therapist; the application guides on the following pages are designed to refresh your memory after you have been taught by the therapist in self-bandaging techniques.

The following guide for upper and lower extremity lymphedema self-bandaging include basic and easy to follow techniques, and do not include all materials and techniques used by your lymphedema therapist. The overall pressure in self-bandaging is much lighter than the one used in phase 1 of the treatment; however, a compression gradient, which means higher pressure on the lower end of the extremity, and lower pressure on top, must still be maintained to achieve the desired results.

The materials and the application sequences may have to be adjusted to your individual situation, including any physical limitations that may be present. You can review these techniques with your lymphedema therapist, who will modify and/or exclude/add certain techniques and materials if necessary.

Materials used in self-bandaging:

- Appropriate skin moisturizer
- Tubular stockinette in the appropriate size
- Gauze bandages 6cm (about 2.5 inches)
- Synthetic padding bandages 10cm, or 15cm (4 or 6 inches)
- Short-stretch bandages in 6, 8, and 10cm widths (2.5, 3, or 4 inches). No "ACE" bandages!
- Tape (masking tape)
- Scissors

The specific materials needed for upper and lower extremity bandaging are listed with the instructions that follow.

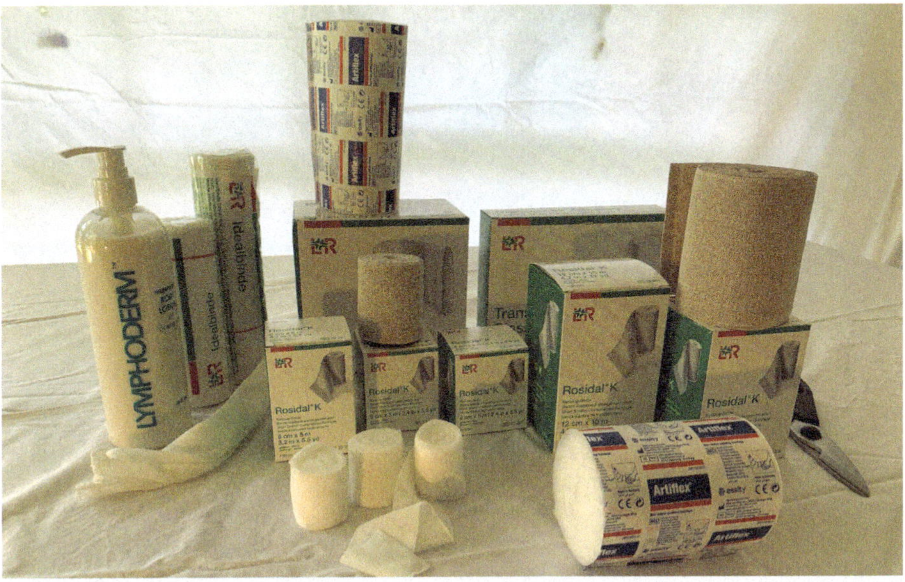

Fig. 3.49 Materials used in self-bandaging

Bandage material is available from a number of online retailers; it is best to discuss your specific needs with your therapist.

Short-stretch bandage brands include Rosidal (Lohmann&Rauscher), Comprilan (Beiersdorf – BSN) and others.

Padding bandages commonly used are Cellona (Lohmann&Rauscher), Artiflex (Beiersdorf – BSN) and others.

Gauze cotton bandages include Elastomull (Beiersdorf–BSN), Mollelast or Transelast (Lohmann&Rauscher) and others.

Tubular stockinette is available as TG (Lohmann&Rauscher), or Tricofix (Beiersdorf – BSN) and others.

Note: Metal clips that come with short-stretch bandages must not be used since they can cause injury to the skin. Instead of clips, tape is used; regular masking tape is appropriate and less expensive than medical tape.

Upper Extremity Self-Bandaging

Materials needed in addition to skin lotion, tubular stockinette and tape:

- 1-2 4cm or 6cm gauze bandages
- 1-2 10cm padding bandages
- 1 6cm short-stretch bandage
- 2-3 10cm or 12cm short-stretch bandages

Gauze bandages and short-stretch bandages are generally applied with 30-40% of stretch, which means that the bandage is pulled to increase its length by about 30-40% during the application. Bandages are applied with a 50% overlap with each layer, which means that each previous layer should be covered about 50% with the next layer of bandages.

1. Apply skin lotion (Fig. 3.50).

2. Apply the tubular stockinette to the arm and allow for about 6 inches extra length on top of the arm. Once the stockinette is on the arm, make a fist and cut the stockinette just below your fist so your arm and hand are covered. Then cut a small hole to allow the thumb to slide through to keep the stockinette in place (Fig. 3.51).

3. Finger bandages: Go around your wrist once without any pull to the gauze in order to anchor it, then continue to wrap each finger with the appropriate stretch (30-40%) and overlap (about 50%). Spread your fingers slightly with the palm facing down and go around each finger 2-3 times; once you are done with one finger, go around the top of your hand before you start with the next finger, so the bandages stay in place. It doesn't matter which finger is bandaged first (Figs. 3.52-3.54).

Note: you can support your arm with a pillow or similar while applying the finger bandages; don't apply full circular turns when anchoring the gauze around the top of your hand between each finger application; don't start or end at a finger; apply tape once you are finished, or tuck the end of the gauze bandage under the previous layers.

4. Apply padding bandage(s) from the hand all the way up to the axilla without any pull on the bandage; overlap by about 50% (Figs. 3.55, 3.56). Make sure the stockinette is pulled all the way up prior to placing the padding bandages; don't use tape with padding bandages, it will damage them. They usually stay in place; you can also tuck the end of the bandage under the previous layer.

5. Start with the first 6cm short-stretch bandage with a loose, no-pull turn around the wrist to anchor it, then proceed to apply the bandage around the hand twice with slightly spread fingers and 30-40% stretch so the hand is covered to the knuckles. From there continue to apply the bandage with stretch and appropriate overlap on the forearm until it is used up. Use tape to affix the end of the short-stretch bandage (Figs. 3.57, 3.58).

6. The next short-stretch bandage (10 or 12cm) is applied in the opposite direction of the first bandage (Fig. 3.59) and starts on the wrist. From there, apply the bandage with stretch and overlap up the arm with the elbow slightly bent. This bandage usually ends at or above the elbow; apply tape to the end of the bandage once it is used up.

7. Apply a third 10 or 12cm bandage, starting below the elbow, to complete the arm all the way up to the axilla and apply tape to secure the bandage (Fig. 3.60). The overlap of the tubular bandage is folded over the last bandage to protect it from perspiration.

In some cases two short-stretch bandages may be sufficient for coverage, depending on the volume and length of the arm, in other cases a forth bandage may be necessary.

Once you completed the bandage, check for an appropriate pressure gradient going up the arm. Bandages should never cause pain, your fingers should not turn blue or red, nor should they feel numb or cold.

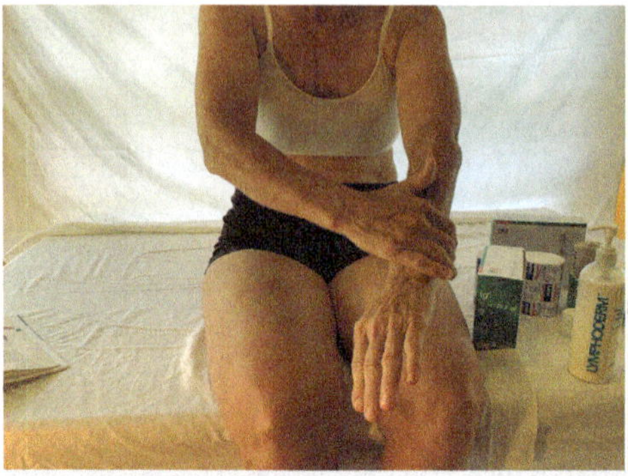

Fig. 3.50

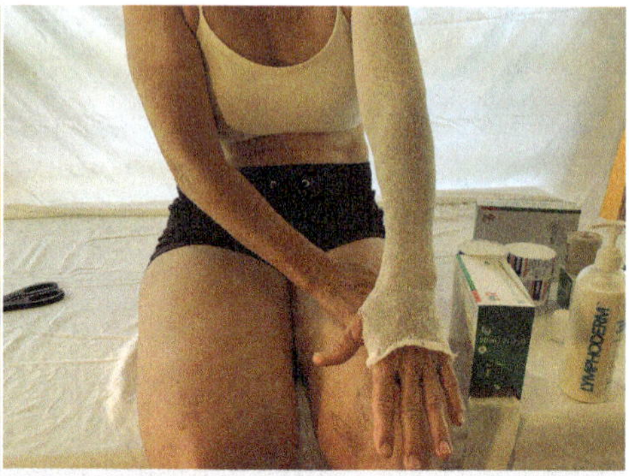

Fig. 3.51

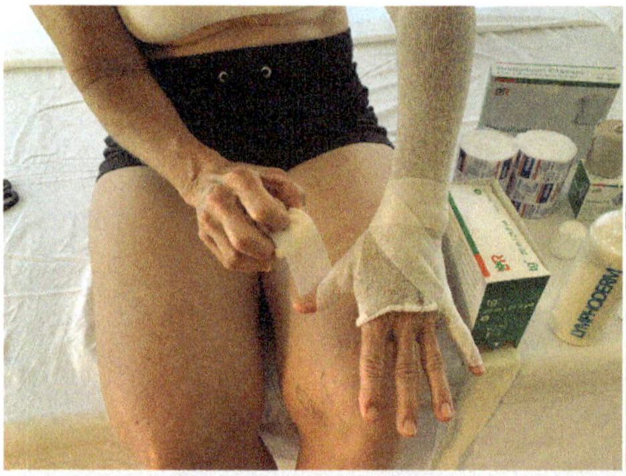

Fig. 3.52

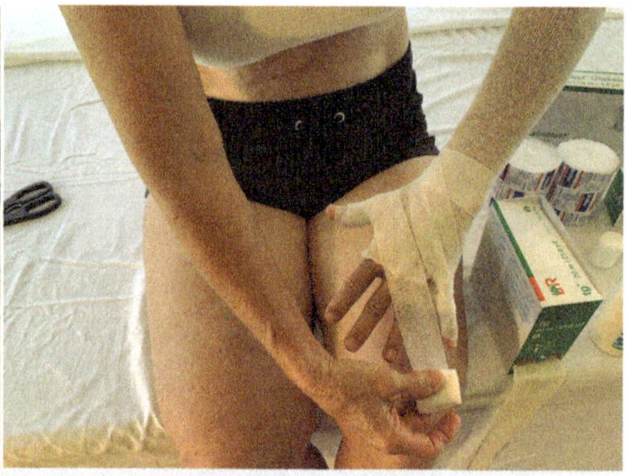
Fig. 3.53

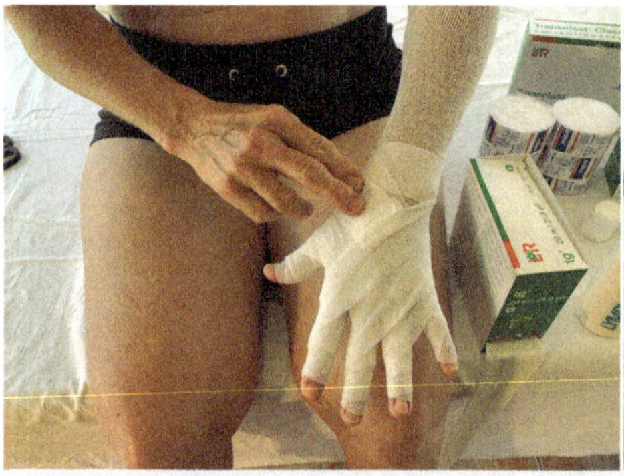
Fig. 3.54

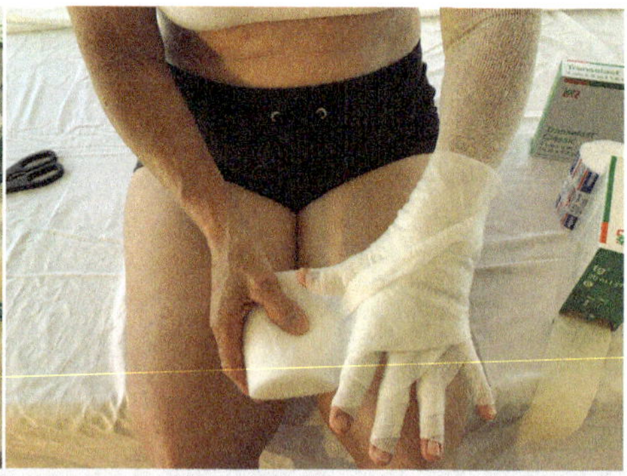
Fig. 3.55

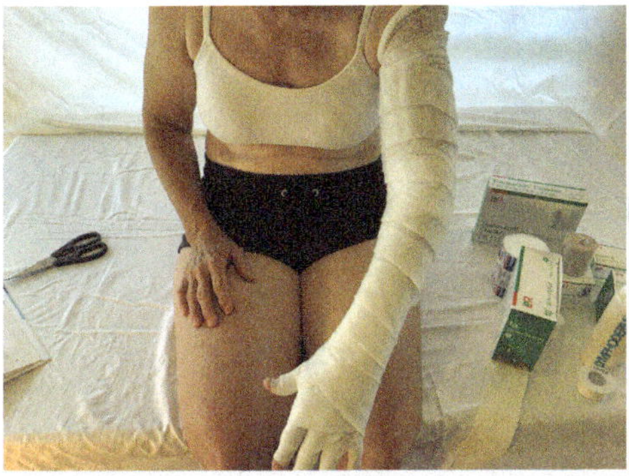

Fig. 3.56

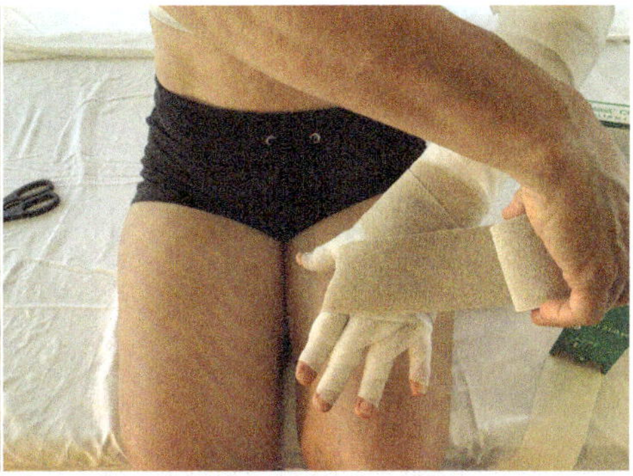

Fig. 3.57

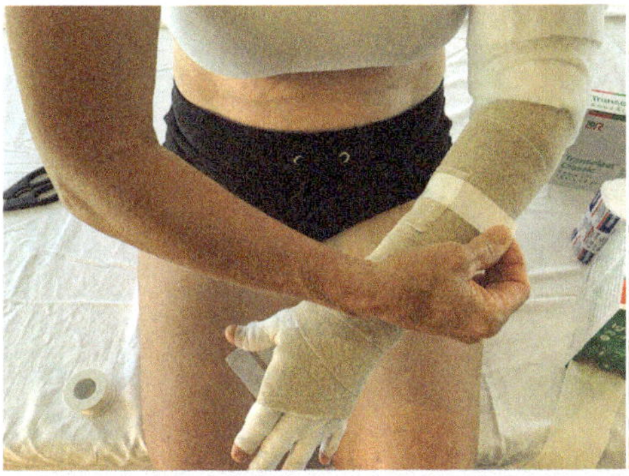

Fig. 3.58

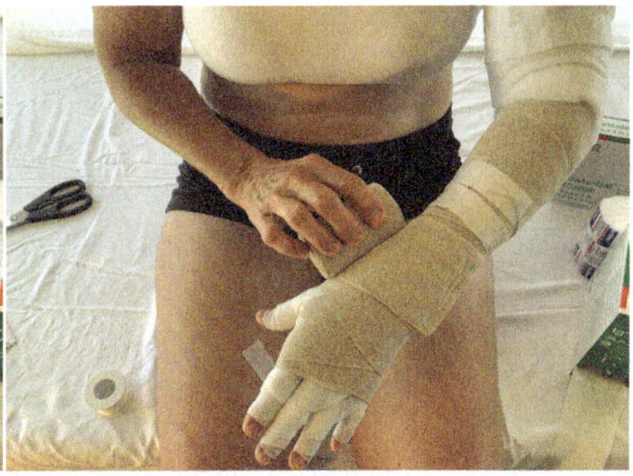

Fig. 3.59

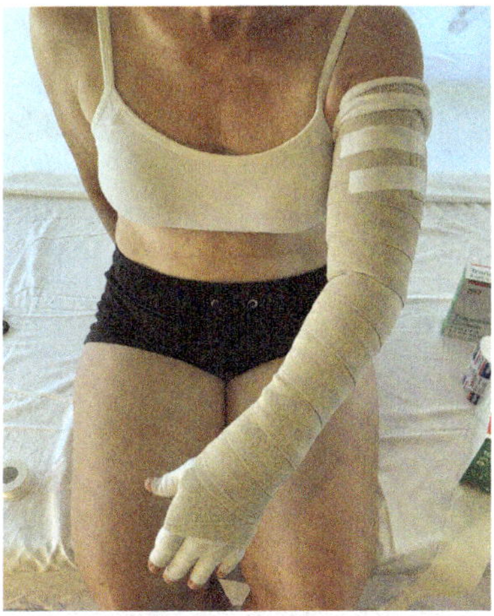

Fig. 3.60

Lower Extremity Self-Bandaging

Materials needed in addition to skin lotion, tubular stockinette and tape:

- 1-2 4cm, or 6cm gauze bandages
- 3-4 10 or 15cm padding bandages
- 1 8cm short-stretch bandage
- 3-5 10cm or 12cm short-stretch bandages

Gauze bandages and short-stretch bandages are generally applied with 30-40% of stretch, which means that the bandage is pulled to increase its length by about 30-40% during the application. Bandages are applied with a 50% overlap with each layer, which means that each previous layer should be covered about 50% with the next layer of bandages.

1. Apply skin lotion.

2. Put the tubular stockinette on the leg and allow for about 6 inches extra length on top of the leg. Once the stockinette is applied to the leg, cut the stockinette just below your toes and fold it over so your foot and leg are completely covered. (Fig. 3.61).

3. If toe bandages are necessary – see next step, if not, ignore.

Use a 4cm gauze bandage (you may also use a 6cm gauze and fold it in half) and wrap it around your foot above the toes once without any pull to the gauze in order to anchor it, then continue to wrap each toe, starting with the big toe with the appropriate stretch (30-40%) and overlap (about 50%). Spread your toes slightly and go around each toe 2-3 times; once you are done with one toe, go around the top of your foot before you start with the next toe, so the gauze stays in place. The little toe does not need to be bandaged, since it rarely is swollen (Figs. 3.62-3.64).

4. Apply padding bandage(s) from the foot all the way up to the groin without any pull on the bandage; overlap by about 50% (Figs. 3.65, 3.66). Make sure the stockinette is pulled all the way up the leg prior to placing the padding

bandages; don't use tape with padding bandages, it will damage them. They usually stay in place; you can tuck the end of the bandage under the previous layer.

5. Start with the first 8cm short-stretch bandage with a loose, no-pull turn around the foot above the toes to anchor it, then proceed to apply the bandage around the foot twice with 30-40% stretch and around 50% overlap so the foot is covered to the beginning of the toes. From there continue to apply the bandage with stretch and appropriate overlap across the top of the ankle and continue around the back of the ankle and over the top of the foot so the bandages form and X pattern. Your ankle should be in 70-90 degrees of flexion, which makes the application easier. Continue with this crisscross fashion around your ankle until it is covered, and proceed to the lower leg until the first bandage is used up (Figs. 3.67 to 3.69).

6. The next short-stretch bandage (10 or 12cm) is applied in the opposite direction of the first bandage (Fig. 3.69) and starts just above the ankle. From there, apply the bandage with stretch and overlap up the lower leg with the knee slightly bent. This bandage usually ends at or above the knee; apply tape to the end of the bandage once it is used up.

7. Apply the next short-stretch bandage (10 or 12cm) just below the knee and continue to wrap the leg over the knee and to the thigh until this bandage is used up (Fig. 3.70). You can apply this bandage either sitting, or standing up.

8. The final short-stretch bandage (12cm or wider) is applied to the thigh, starting above the knee and wrap all the way up to the groin and apply tape to secure the bandage (Fig. 3.71). The overlap of the tubular bandage is folded over the last bandage.

In some cases, an additional short-stretch bandage may be necessary, depending on the volume and length of the leg.

Once you completed the bandage, check for an appropriate pressure gradient going up the leg. Bandages should never cause pain, your toes should not turn blue or red, nor should they feel numb or cold.

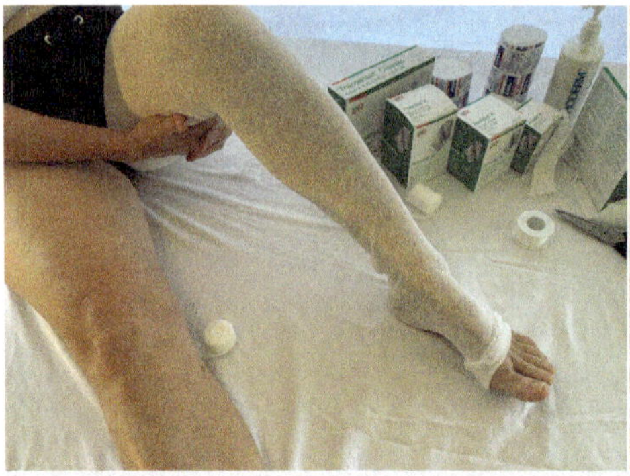

Fig. 3.61

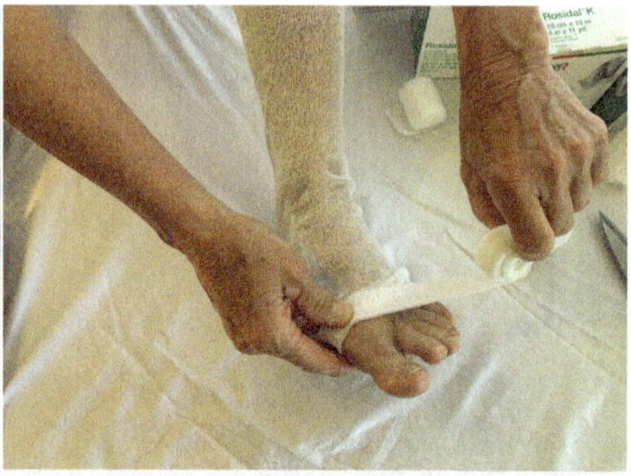

Fig. 3.62

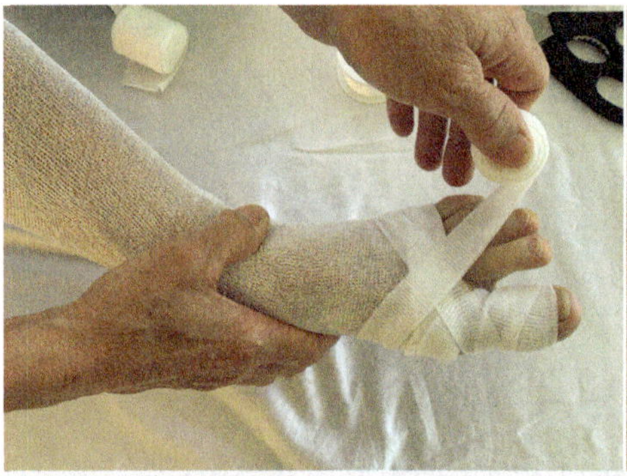

Fig. 3.63

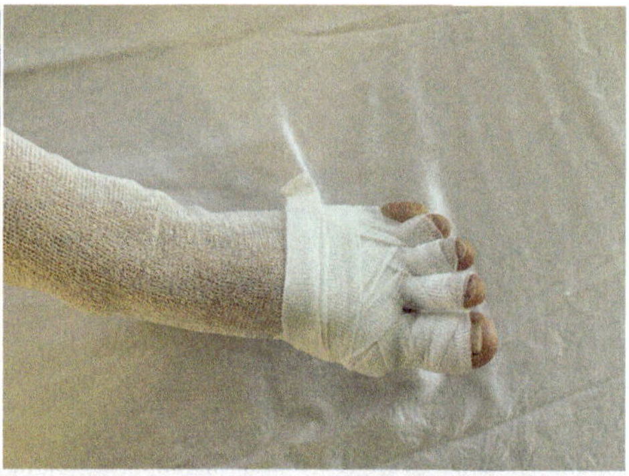

Fig. 3.64

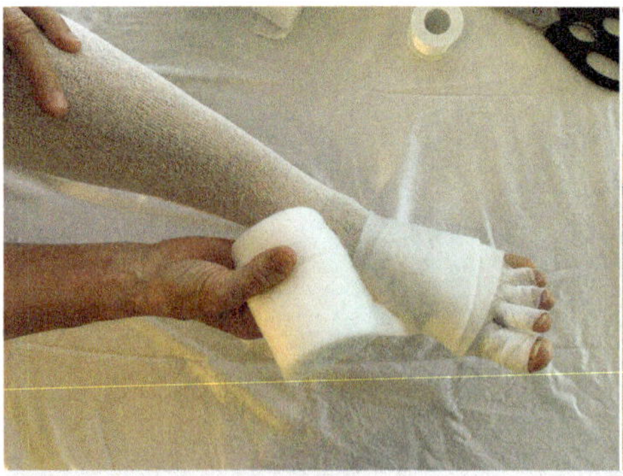

Fig. 3.65

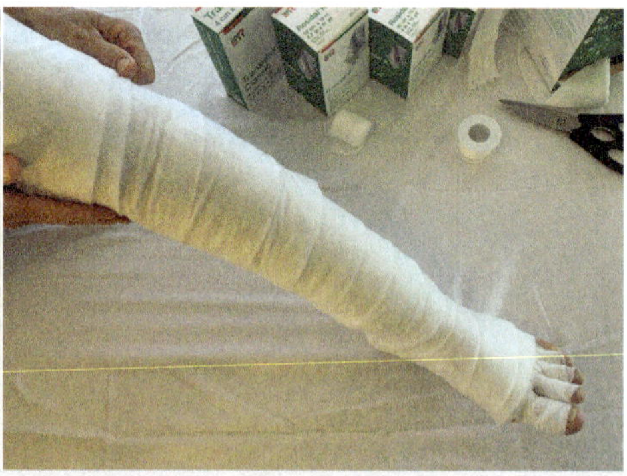

Fig. 3.66

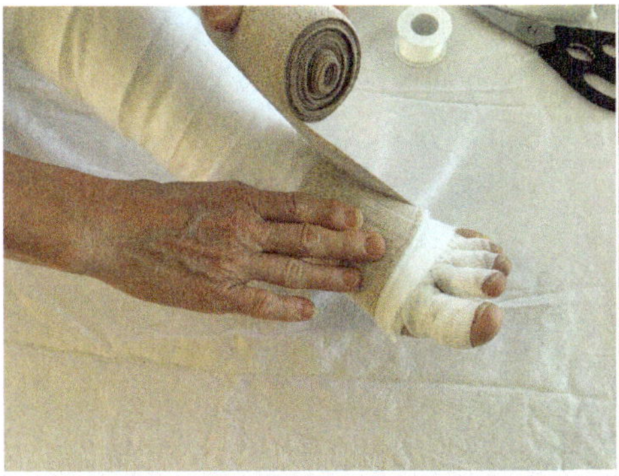

Fig. 3.67

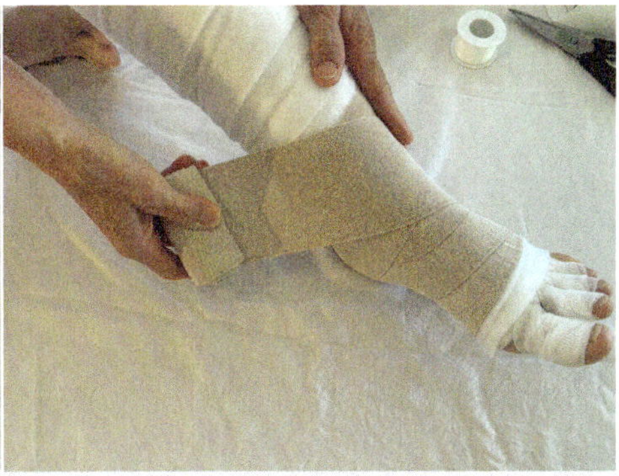

Fig. 3.68

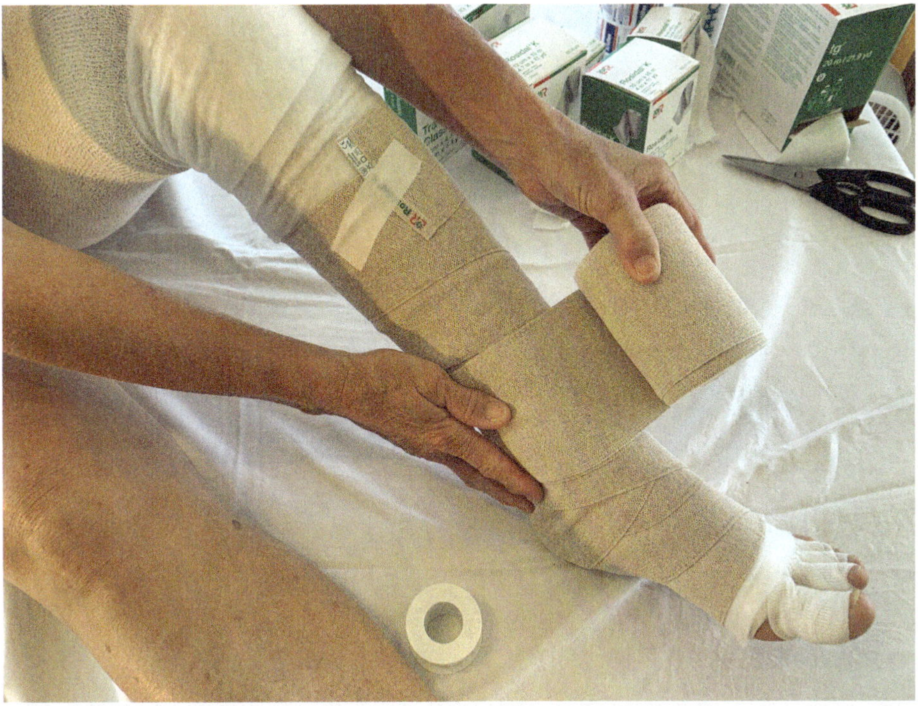

Fig. 3.69

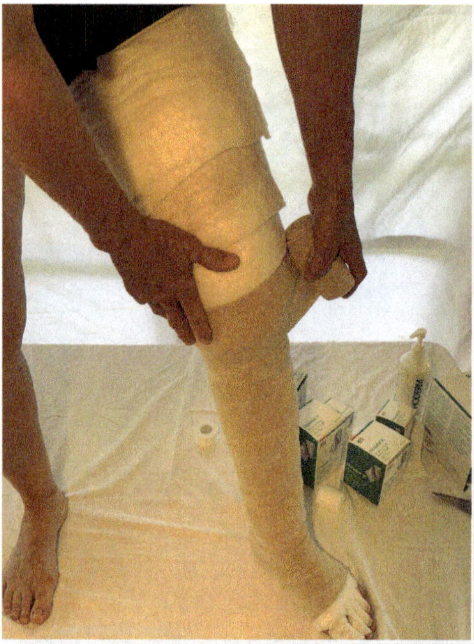

Fig. 3.70

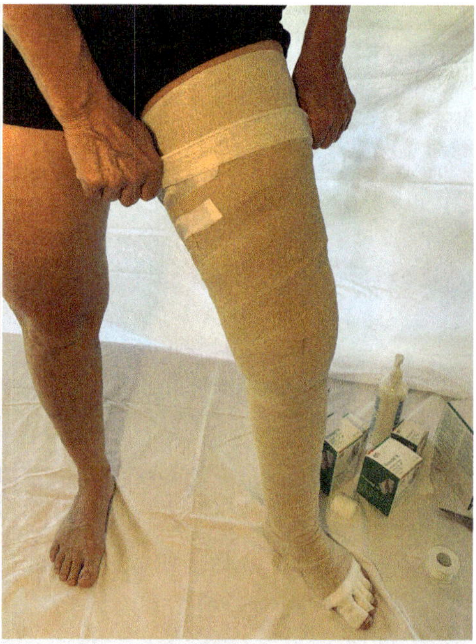

Fig. 3.71

Instead of padding bandages to distribute the pressure applied by the short-stretch bandages, bandage liners may be used (Figs. 3.5 a, b). These liners are applied underneath the short-stretch bandages and are filled with foam particles and "built-in" channels to help direct the flow of lymph.

Compression in phase 2 of CDT can also be managed using alternate compression devices. These products are easy to put on and can be adjusted for fluctuations in shape and size using non-elastic and adjustable bands with velcro closures. Alternative compression materials are applied on top of padding, and replace short-stretch bandages. These devices, or wraps require the measurements be taken by the lymphedema therapist or certified fitter (Figs. 3.3; 3.10 a-c; 3.11 a-c).

Bandage liners and alternate compression devices work well, but are a more costly alternative to regular self-bandaging.

3.6.3 Exercises

A balanced exercise program plays an important part in reducing and maintaining the swelling in lymphedema, and presents a vital tool for patients to continue with normal activities of daily living.

Patients who have lymphedema profoundly benefit from regular exercises, which assist in weight control, improved strength, endurance, decreased severity and prevention of lymphedema related symptoms, such as restricted joint mobility, and improve immune function, mood and energy level. Exercises also play an important role in supporting venous and lymphatic return to the blood circulatory system, which assists in decongestion and helps to maintain the reduction of lymphedema.

Exercises performed with the certified lymphedema therapist in the intensive phase of CDT generally involve simple decongestive, or remedial exercises, consisting of hip, knee and ankle flexes, shoulder shrugs, shoulder movements and elbow bends, etc., which are best performed with the compression bandages in place.

Once phase 1 of CDT is completed, and the patients are fitted for a compression garment, patients can return to most of the exercise routines performed prior to developing lymphedema. Almost all exercise routines can be adjusted and modified to account for certain restrictions due to the presence of lymphedema; some exercises require more caution, especially if injury is a concern. Examples include sports including a racket (tennis, squash, golf) for patients with lymphedema of the arm, or extensive running, kickboxing, or step-aerobics for those affected by lymphedema of the leg.

Beneficial activities include stretching and mobility exercises (Yoga), aerobic exercises, such as walking, swimming, easy biking, as well as breathing and decongestive exercises. These modalities are described in more detail on previous pages under Exercises.

Lymphedema patients were regularly advised in the past to protect their extremity from overuse following surgery, especially concerning resistive and aerobic exercises. Newer research studies show ample evidence that exercises are not linked to the worsening of lymphedema symptoms, and are beneficial if performed with slow progression in intensity and under initial supervision of a trained health care professional [8-11].

Yoga

Several studies [29-31] indicate that the benefits of yoga can have very beneficial effects for patients affected by lymphedema of the arms and legs. Yoga can be easily adapted to the individual's particular health status, abilities and limitations, and therefore may be preferable to more strenuous forms of exercise for some patients. In addition to increasing flexibility, muscle strength and range of motion, yoga beneficially impacts diaphragmatic breathing, and increases venous and lymphatic circulation, both important aspects in the management of lymphedema.

The downward and upward movement of the diaphragm in deep abdominal breathing is an essential component for the sufficient return of lymphatic fluid back to the bloodstream; movement of the diaphragm, combined with the outward and inward movements of the abdomen, rib cage, and lower back, also promotes general well-being, relaxation, peristalsis and return of venous blood back to the heart. The controlled breathing exercises performed in yoga promote lymph flow by strengthening the diaphragm and its movement. Resting and paying attention to the breath between yoga poses helps the body to relax from the previous pose, and prepare for the next pose without strain.

There are many different forms of yoga; some are fast-paced and intense, others are gentle and relaxing. The intensity level varies with the type of yoga. Techniques like "Hatha" and "Iyengar" yoga are gentle and slow; "Bikram", "Hot" and "Power" yoga are faster, more challenging techniques and should be avoided by those affected by lymphedema. More advanced poses, and most of the inverted poses should be avoided by individuals affected by lymphedema of the arm, including headstand (too much weight on the arms and neck), shoulder stand (too much weight and pressure on the neck and shoulders), and downward facing dog (too much weight on the arms).

The gentler forms of yoga, combined with breathing exercises, are preferable for patients with lymphedema of the upper and lower extremities.

Examples of different types of yoga:

Hatha: This form is most often associated with yoga and is one of the most popular styles; it combines a series of most of the basic movements of yoga and focuses on breath controlled exercises. The breathing exercises are followed by a series of yoga postures, which are generally held longer than in other yoga variations, and end with a resting period.

The traditional poses may need to be adapted to the individual's capabilities. In a yoga class situation, patients should ask the instructor to modify the pose if necessary; patients exercising on their own with a book or video may try going into the pose only half-way or skipping it altogether.

Simple lateral and twisting poses, along with basic forward and backward bending poses are most recommended for lymphedema yoga. Most yoga classes taught in the West are different variations of Hatha yoga.

Iyengar: Iyengar is a very meticulous style of yoga, with great attention paid to finding the proper alignment in a pose. In a typical Iyengar class, poses are held much longer than with other forms of yoga. Typical for this form of yoga is the use of props, such as blocks, belts, bolsters, chairs and blankets to assist the body to move into the proper alignment and accommodate any limitation, injuries, tightness or structural imbalances the patient may have.

Vinyasa: This is also a very popular style of yoga practice, which involves synchronizing the breath with the continuous performance of a series of postures that flow smoothly into one another. Vinyasa classes are known for their fluid, movement-intensive practices. Vinyasa instructors arrange their classes to smoothly transition from pose to pose, and often play music. The intensity of the practice is similar to Ashtanga.

Ashtanga: This form is a more challenging, physically demanding variation of yoga that follows a specific, typically fast-paced, sequence of a series of postures, all of which are linked to breathing. Ashtanga is like Vinyasa yoga, as each style links every movement to a breath. The difference is that Ashtanga always performs the exact same poses in the exact same order.

Power Yoga: A faster and high intensity practice, which is more fitness based. In addition to other benefits of yoga, this variation builds muscular strength and increases stamina, but is physically very demanding.

Bikram: This form is also known as "hot yoga," and consists of a copyrighted series of 26 challenging poses performed in a room heated to 104 degrees Fahrenheit (40 degrees Celsius) with a humidity level of 40%. Bikram classes always follow the same sequence, and classes run over a period of 90 minutes. This form of yoga is physically highly challenging.

Hot Yoga: Hot yoga is very similar to Bikram. The main differences include temperature; the room is generally heated to about 80-100 degrees Fahrenheit. Yoga postures vary within different classes and are not restricted to 26 poses; the duration of a class is typically 60 minutes.

The universal caution for any exercise "don't strain" is crucial for those concerned with the goal of preventing the onset of, and those affected by lymphedema. The focus for those who consider the practice of yoga should be on increasing lymph flow through postures and breathing, stress and pain relief, increased flexibility and strength, improved balance and well-being.

Based on the information above, the most appropriate variations of yoga for lymphedema patients include Hatha, Iyengar and moderate variations of Vinyasa. These forms are gentle, relatively simple, focus on breathing and are still physically challenging but not overwhelming. Additional benefits of yoga include weight management, improved strength, cardiovascular conditioning (lowering blood pressure and resting heart rate, increasing endurance and improving oxygen uptake during exercise), inner calm, support of a healthy life style and encouragement to self-care.

Individuals who have lymphedema should always wear their compression garments or bandages during yoga exercises to support and increase lymphatic and venous return. Should any pain develop during yoga exercises it is recommended that patients take a rest, elevate the arm or leg, and focus on breathing exercises.

Beneficial yoga poses for lymphedema:

Elevated legs up the wall: This exercise is performed laying on the back on the floor and raising your legs up against a wall. While sitting, bring one side of your body close to a wall, swivel your legs up the wall and lay your upper body on the floor. Lift your buttocks up off the floor a few inches and place a blanket or bolster under your tailbone.

Half standing forward bend: While standing with your feet hip width apart, bend your body forward to a horizontal position while stretching your hands out in front of you. Another option is to place your hands on a chair or a table with your arms stretched out, the hands rest on the chair or the table.

Simple arm and hand movements: Can be performed sitting in a chair or cross-legged on the floor. Arms are raised, ideally holding a band, over the head while inhaling. The arms are lowered, or extended behind the head while exhaling.

A description of beneficial and easy to perform decongestive exercises for lymphedema are listed on the following pages. Common for all these exercises is the involvement of the joint and muscle pumps, which assist lymphatic and venous return. Please follow the general rules for exercising with lymphedema and wear your compression bandages or garments while conducting lymphedema exercises; an older, worn compression garment can be worn when exercising in the water.

Exercises for Upper Extremity Lymphedema

Wear comfortable clothing; exercises are ideally performed sitting on a stool, chair, or table, or standing, and following the self-MLD treatment protocol; session should last about 10-15 minutes. Aim to conduct the exercises in a controlled and slow manner with the muscles relaxing between individual exercises with 3-5 (or more) repetitions each. Exercises should never cause pain or discomfort.

Begin with your neck, then proceed to the shoulder area and move down the arm.

Neck:

1. Bend your neck slowly to each side, aiming to touch the shoulder with your ear without shrugging the shoulder (Fig. 3.72).

2. Slowly turn your head to each side, trying to look over your shoulder (Fig. 3.73).

Shoulder and arm; stand or sit with your arms relaxed by your side:

3. Shrug both shoulders; inhale while trying to bring your shoulders to your ears, and exhale while returning to the starting position (Fig. 3.74).

4. Shoulder rolls; rotate both shoulders alternating, or at the same time (Fig. 3.75).

5. Lift both arms to the side, either alternating, or at the same time. Inhale as you lift the arms to shoulder height, and exhale while returning to the starting position (Fig. 3.76).

6. Bring your arm with lymphedema straight to the front up to shoulder height while breathing in, and lower the arm to the starting position when breathing out (Fig. 3.77).

7. Sideways stretch; try touching your opposite ear with the fingers of your lymphedema arm, then stretch your torso to the opposite side so you feel a stretch along the side of the torso on your lymphedema side. Inhale while you stretch, breathe out when returning to the starting position (Fig. 3.78).

8. Stretch out your lymphedema arm to the front, as if picking something, make a fist and return to the starting position. Inhale as you move to the front, exhale while moving back (Fig. 3.79).

9. Perform breaststrokes, as if swimming, as far as possible to the front while inhaling. Move the arm back while exhaling (Figs. 3.80, 3.81).

10. Bend both arms at the elbow and bring your hands as close as possible to your shoulders while inhaling (biceps curl). Exhale while returning to the starting position (Fig. 3.82).

11. Extend your lymphedema arm to the front with the palm facing downward and bend your wrist while breathing in; breathe out when you return the hand to the starting point (Fig. 3.83).

Hand and fingers:

12. Hold the palm of your lymphedema arm in front of you with the palm facing up; move the thumb and index fingers together so they touch. Repeat touching each finger with your thumb, opening the hand completely between each finger touch (Fig. 3.84).

13. Make a fist while inhaling, and open the hand breathing out. You may also perform this exercise with a soft ball and with your arm elevated (Fig. 3.85).

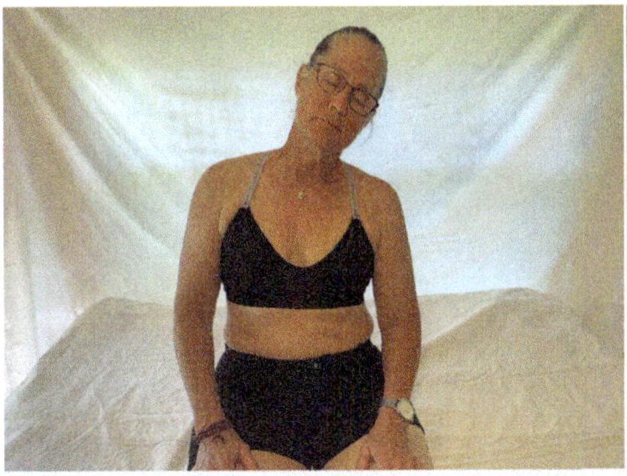
Fig. 3.72

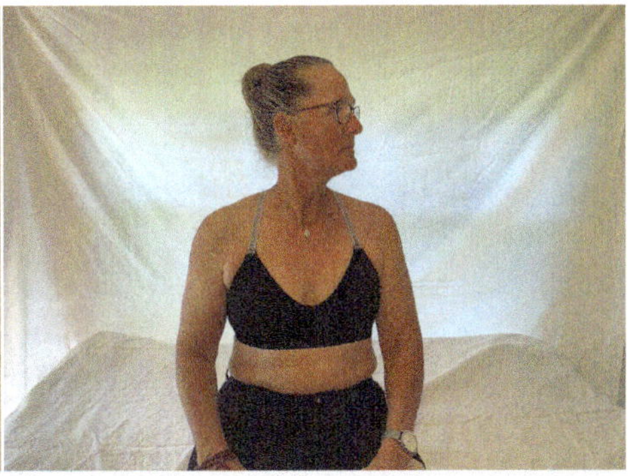
Fig. 3.73

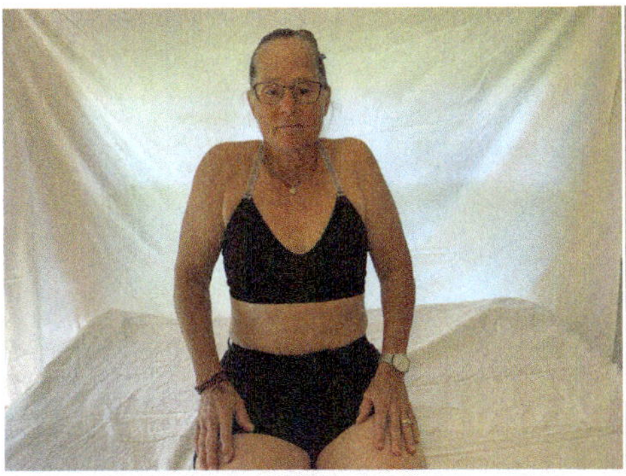
Fig. 3.74

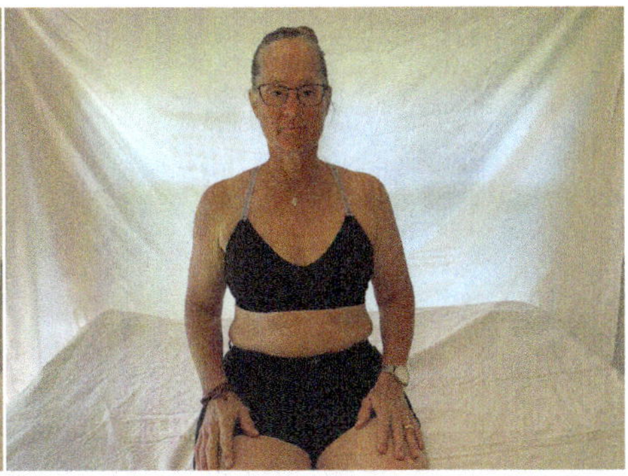
Fig. 3.75

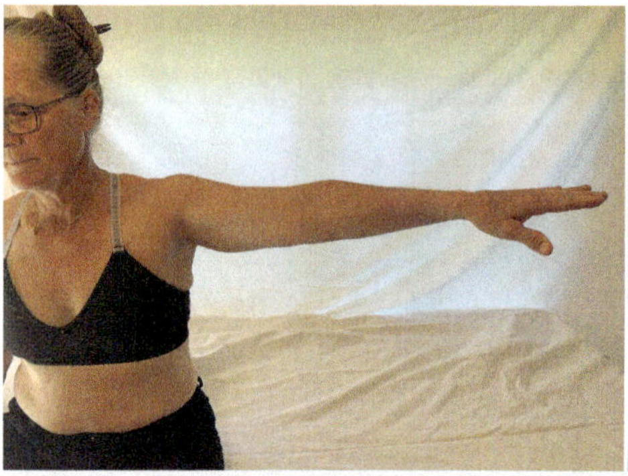

Fig. 3.76

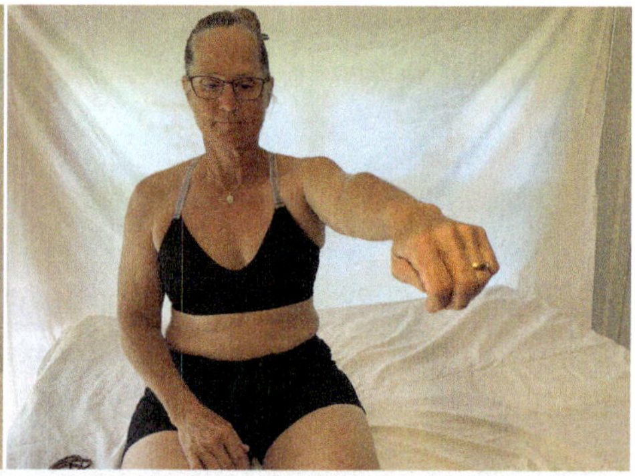

Fig. 3.77

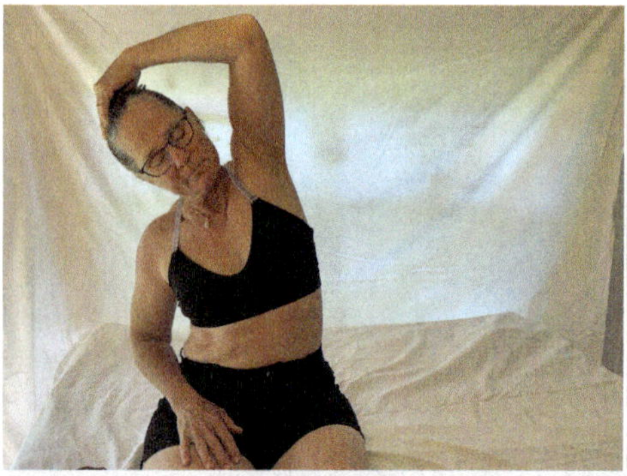

Fig. 3.78

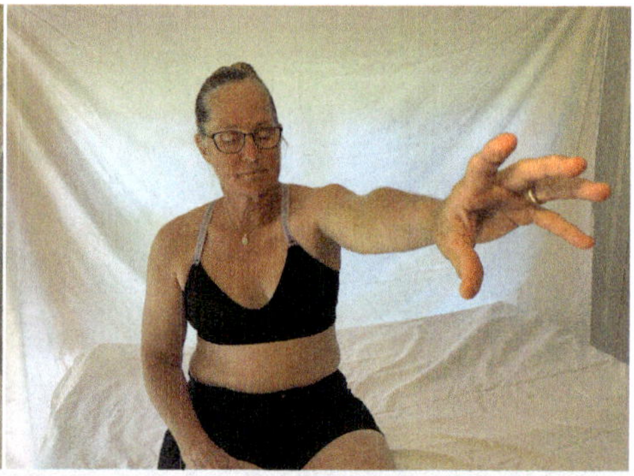

Fig. 3.79

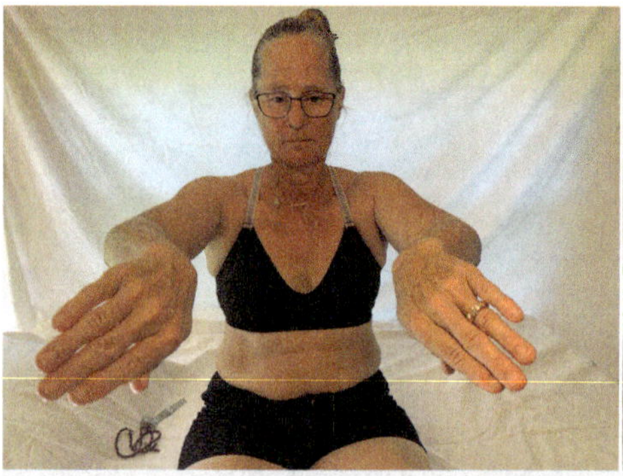

Fig. 3.80

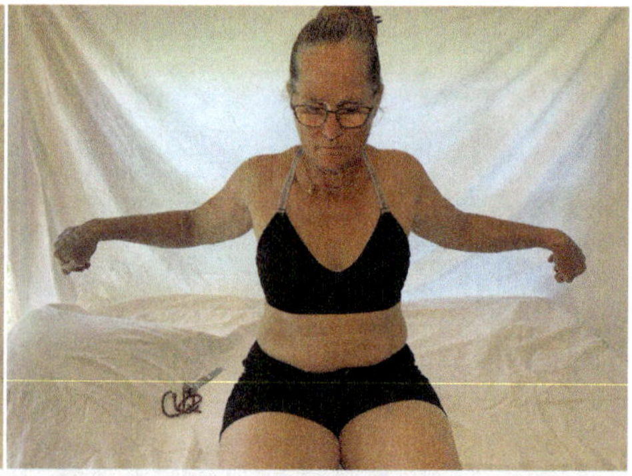

Fig. 3.81

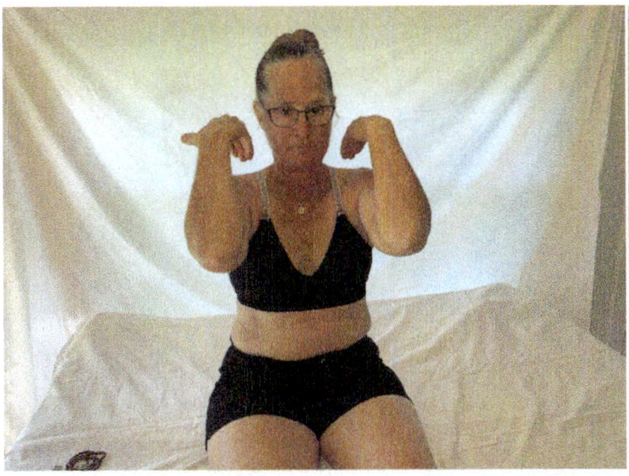

Fig. 3.82

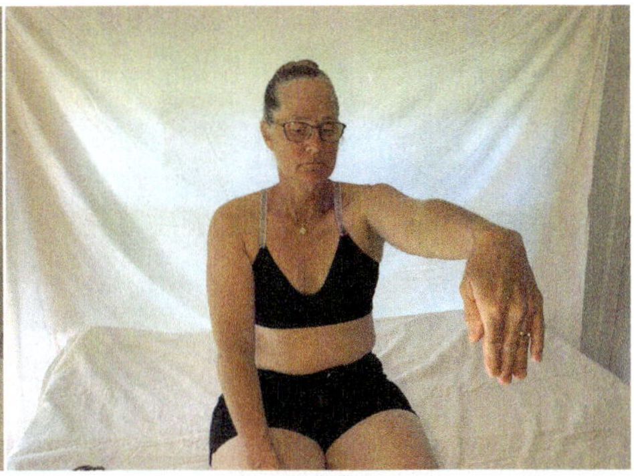

Fig. 3.83

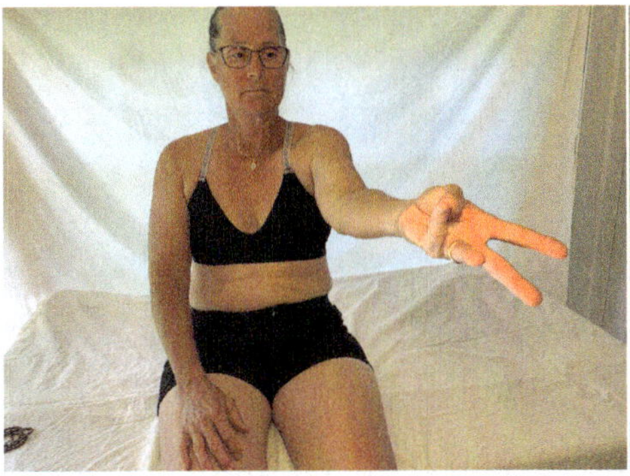

Fig. 3.84

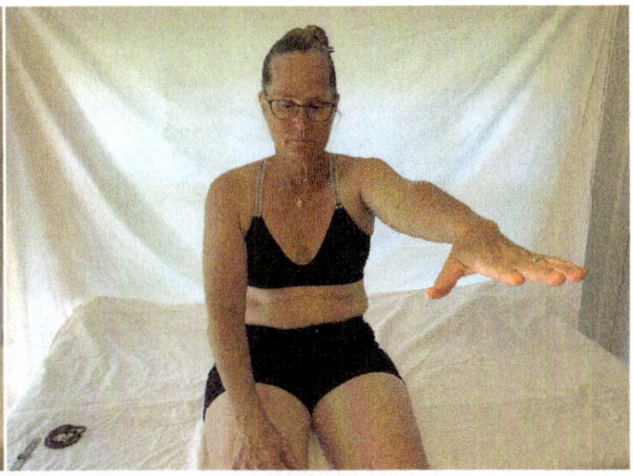

Fig. 3.85

Exercises for Lower Extremity Lymphedema

Wear comfortable clothing; exercises are ideally performed standing, or lying supine, preferably on a mat providing some firmness. However, leg exercises can also be conducted sitting on a stool, or table. Ideally, exercises are performed following the self-MLD treatment protocol; session should last about 10-15 minutes. Aim to conduct the exercises in a controlled and slow manner with the muscles relaxing between individual exercises with 3-5 (or more) repetitions each. Exercises should never cause pain or discomfort.

Begin with your neck, then proceed with abdominal breathing exercises (consult with your therapist for any possible contraindications, such as recent surgery or radiation to the abdominal area, diverticulitis, and others); then continue with the hip and move down the leg.

Neck:

1. Bend your neck slowly to each side, aiming to touch the shoulder with your ear without shrugging the shoulder (Fig. 3.86).

2. Slowly turn your head to each side, trying to look over your shoulder (Fig. 3.87).

3. Abdominal (diaphragmatic) breathing exercises: Inhale through your nose against your hands into the belly, so that you feel your stomach rising against your flat hands. Exhale slowly with your lips pursed and your hands gently following the belly down to your spine and slightly upward into the chest. Repeat 5-10 times. Should you feel dizzy, or if the downward movement causes discomfort, stop (Figs. 3.88, 3.89).

Legs:

4. Elevate your lymphedema leg with the knee flexed towards your torso while exhaling; return to the starting position while breathing in (Fig. 3.90).

5. Bring your straight leg out to the side as you exhale; return to the starting point while inhaling (Fig. 3.91).

6. Move the heel of your leg as close as possible to your buttocks while breathing out, breathe in while going back to the starting position (Fig. 3.92).

7. Lift your lymphedema leg and push with the opposite palm against your knee while exhaling; inhale while going back to the starting point (Fig. 3.93).

8. Rotate the ankle of your lymphedema leg in circles; you can do this exercise either with the heel lifted, or resting on the mat (Fig. 3.94).

9. Flex and extend the ankle of your lymphedema leg; you can do this exercise either with the heel lifted, or resting on the mat (Fig. 3.95).

9. Curl the toes of your lymphedema leg as if you would pick something up with your toes (Fig. 3.96).

10. Spread the toes of your lymphedema leg as far apart as possible (Fig. 3.97).

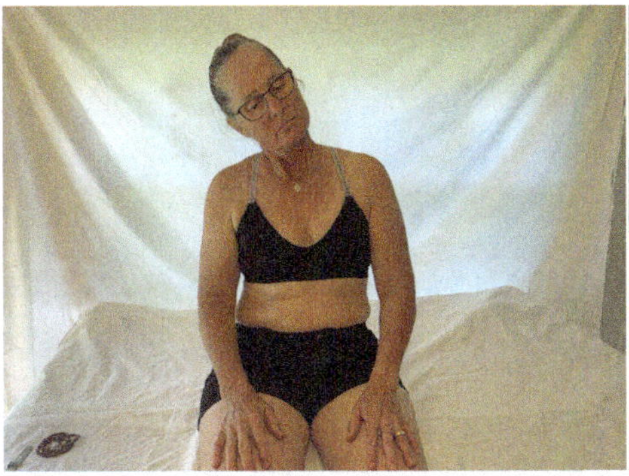

Fig. 3.86

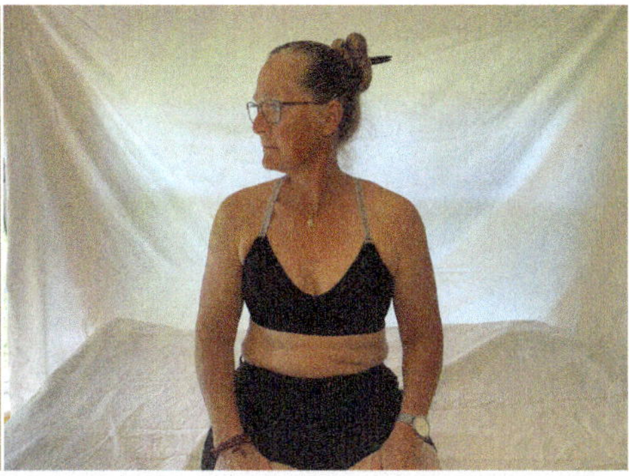

Fig. 3.87

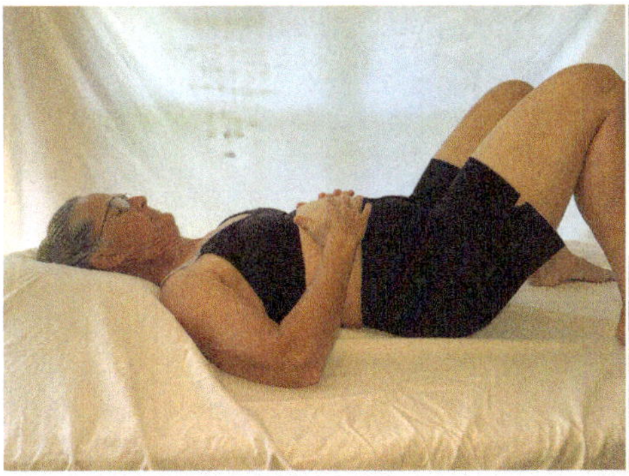

Fig. 3.88

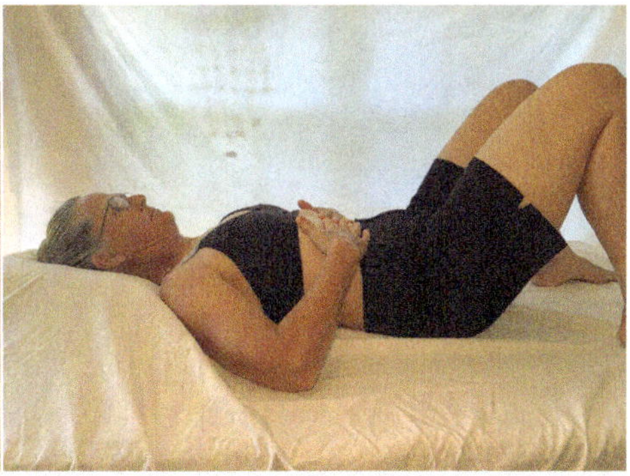

Fig. 3.89

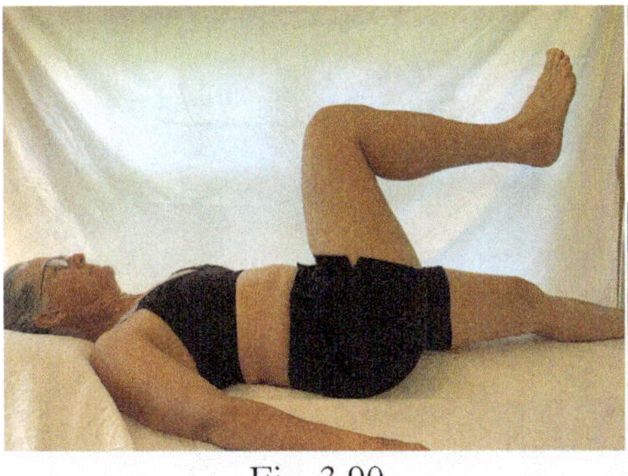

Fig. 3.90

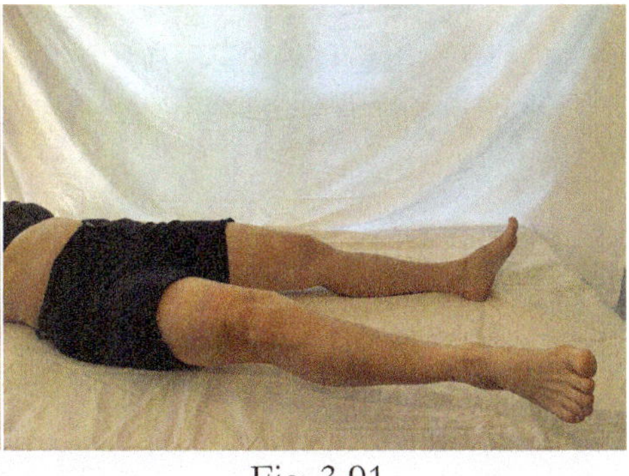

Fig. 3.91

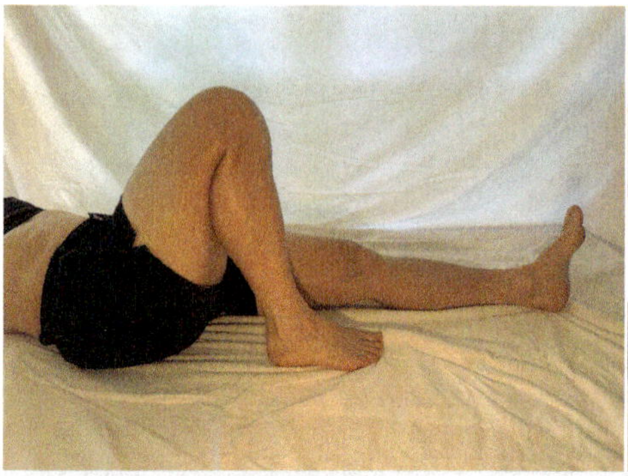

Fig. 3.92

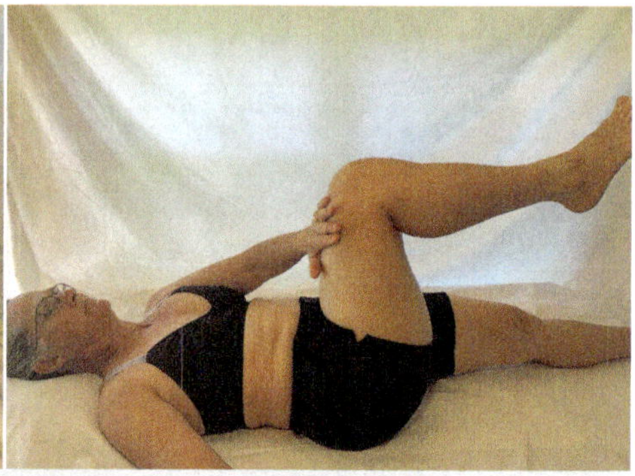

Fig. 3.93

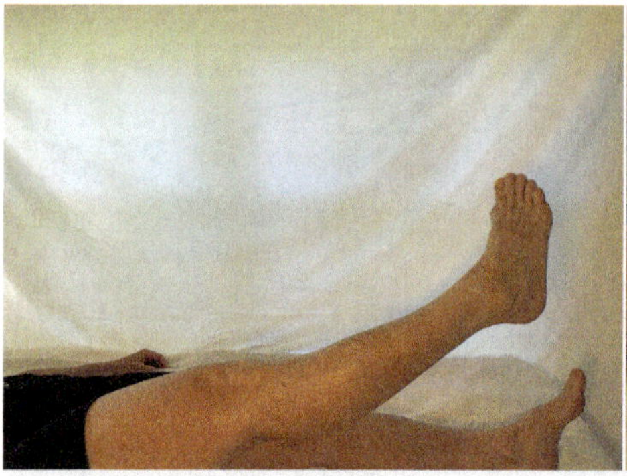

Fig. 3.94

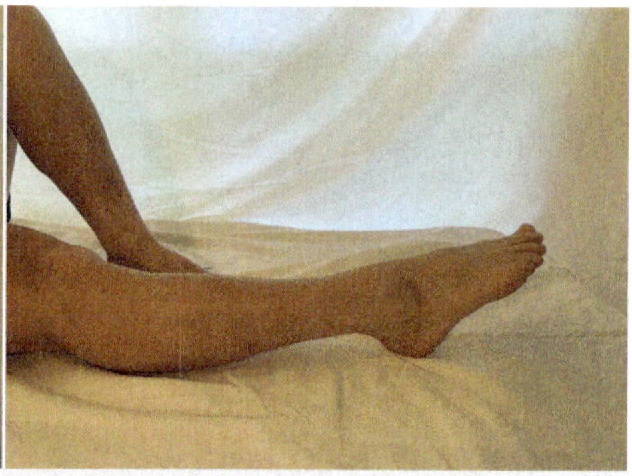

Fig. 3.95

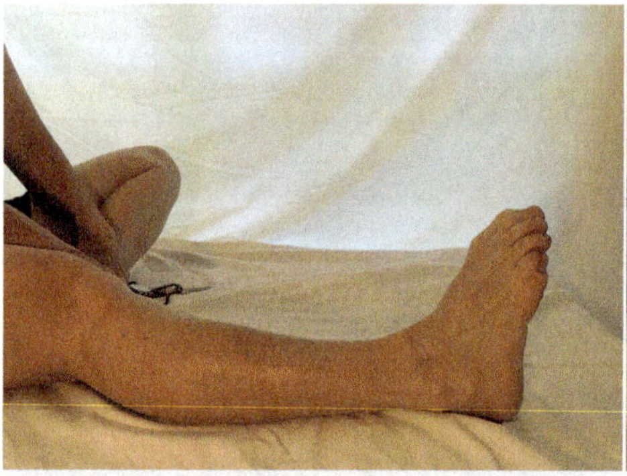

Fig. 3.96

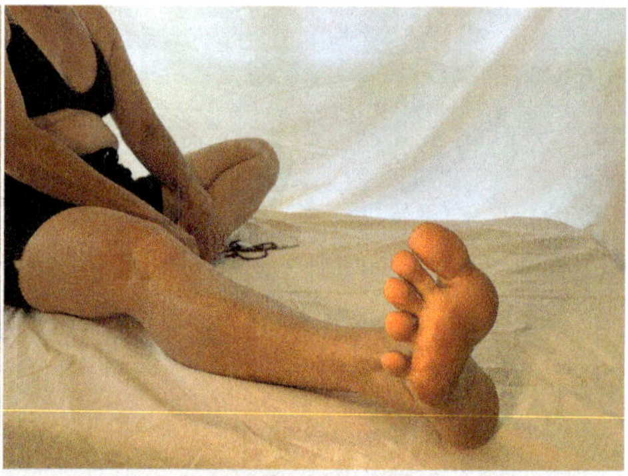

Fig. 3.97

3.7 General Information for Patients with Lymphedema

Lymphedema Risk Reduction

To avoid the onset of lymphedema, health care professionals should follow expert consensus regarding best practices to avoiding lymphedema, or infections in existing lymphedema, and inform patients with breast cancer and other cancers about their risk factors for developing lymphedema [15,36]. There is ample research available on the benefits of patient education for reducing the risk of developing lymphedema following surgery; most research covers the risks of breast cancer related lymphedema [34, 35].

The surgical procedures performed on individuals affected by breast cancer may be mastectomy, partial mastectomy, or lumpectomy. Along with the actual breast surgery for cancer, lymph nodes in the axilla are removed and/ or radiated.

As a result of axillary lymph node clearance, the normal lymphatic drainage from the extremity is impaired, and some patients experience the onset of lymphedema.

Accumulated lymph fluid in the swollen extremity provides a rich culture medium for bacteria, which makes lymphedematous tissues susceptible to infections. Simple injuries and puncture wounds can develop into local or generalized infections that may produce further lymphatic destruction and blockage. To reduce the risk of these postoperative complications, most patients are advised to not have blood pressure readings taken on, intravenous infusions in, or blood samples taken from the arm on the operated side.

Very little published data is available to document the exact risk of lymphedema from performing blood pressure readings, blood draws, and injections on the affected extremity. Lack of research and normal variations in each individual's lymphatic system (numbers or sizes of remaining lymph nodes) make it difficult to quantify personal risk from each triggering factor.

An article published in 2016 in the Journal of Clinical Oncology [32] on risk-reduction practices concluded that risk-reduction practices are overrated and/ or no risk reduction behaviors are needed for lymphedema.

While the article was published in a reputable medical journal reporting on a study from a Harvard-affiliated hospital, there were serious limitations in this study, which also had very a limited number of participants. The study concluded: "Although we cannot affirmatively state that risk-reduction practices have no effect on arm swelling, we hope to generate evidence that brings reasonable doubt to burdensome guidelines and encourage further investigation into non-precautionary behaviors and the risk of lymphedema."

The flawed conclusions drawn from this study were outlined in a response, which was published in the same journal[33]. To be clear, risk reduction behaviors for lymphedema have not been debunked. However, if healthcare providers do not read the entire article critically and concentrate on the one-line synopsis only, they might conclude that reputable journals have shown that risk reduction behaviors are needed any longer for lymphedema.

This presents a problem for patients and puts them in a difficult situation, as they may ask not to have blood pressure measurements, IV's, or blood draws in their at-risk extremity, and be met with resistance from providers that may have read that article.

Research suggests that the risk of complications resulting from blood draws or intravenous injections on the affected extremity is low; however, there is still a risk, which is avoidable.

Not all medical professionals are familiar with the precautions for avoiding lymphedema, so patients must be especially watchful advocates for themselves.

While further research is needed, healthcare professionals are encouraged to minimize the risk of lymphedema by taking blood pressure readings, blood draws and injections on the non-affected limb whenever possible.

In patients with breast cancer on both sides, these procedures should be performed on the leg or the foot. If this is not possible, the procedure should be done on the non-dominant arm. If one side had no lymph node removal, the arm on that side should be used, regardless of whether it is the dominant arm.

In an emergency, however (such as a car accident), or if a medically necessary procedure (such as a CT or MRI) needs to be performed, and an intravenous line must be started, medical professionals must be allowed to do what they need to do to start the intravenous line as soon as possible, even if it would involve the affected extremity.

If a port is present, blood draws should be taken directly from there. In patients with "bad" veins, good hydration and some form of heat (heat pads, warm water) help to dilate the veins prior to cannulation.

Following are some general guidelines to reduce the risk of lymphedema.

Upper Extremity

Certain activities may trigger the onset of lymphedema or may exacerbate the symptoms of existing lymphedema. Individuals affected by primary or secondary lymphedema, and those at risk for developing it (everyone who has undergone lymph node removal and/or radiation treatments) should observe the following precautions, which are based on decades of experience and knowledge of clinical experts in the field of lymphedema management.

Skin Care

- Keep your skin meticulously clean and check frequently for any cracks, infections, or rashes.
- Moisturize your skin daily, especially after taking a shower or bath.
- Use appropriate ointments or lotions.
- Dry your skin thoroughly with a soft towel following a shower or bath; do not scrub.
- If you undergo radiation therapy, apply the ointments recommended by your physician to any radiation redness on your skin and avoid direct exposure to sunlight.
- Avoid cosmetics that irritate the skin.

Clothing, Jewelry, Compression Sleeve, Prosthesis

- Avoid clothing that is too tight, such as bras and sleeves that cause restriction; you should use a comfortable bra with wide and padded shoulder straps.
- Do not wear tight jewelry and avoid elastic bands around your wrist.
- Wear your compression sleeve all day, and if necessary, apply your bandages at night. Use rubber gloves when you put on your compression sleeve. See your certified lymphedema therapist (CLT) at least every six months to check the condition of the garment.
- Discuss with your doctor and/or therapist, what kind of external breast prosthesis is appropriate in your case (heavier silicone or lighter foam).

Avoid any Injuries to the Skin

- Shaving: use an electric razor to remove hair from your armpit or chest; do not use razor blades.
- Nail care: you should keep your fingernails cut short; avoid the use of scissors for cutting your fingernails; do not cut the cuticles. Avoid artificial nails.
- Should you smoke, do not extinguish the cigarette with your affected hand.
- Wear gloves when gardening and playing with your pets (scratches).
- Mosquito bites: wear insect repellents, avoid mosquito-infested areas.
- Injections and blood draw: blood draws and injections on the non-affected limb whenever possible. In patients with breast cancer on both sides, these procedures should be performed on the leg or the foot. If this is not possible, the procedure should be done on the non-dominant arm. If one side had no lymph node removal, the arm on that side should be used, regardless of whether it is the dominant arm. In an emergency, however (such as a car accident), or if a medically necessary procedure (such as a CT or MRI) needs to be performed,

and an intravenous line must be started, medical professionals must be allowed to do what they need to do to start the intravenous line as soon as possible, even if it would involve the affected extremity. If a port is present, blood draws should be taken directly from there.

- Avoid blood pressure to be taken on the affected arm or the arm at risk. Have the clinician use the other arm, or if both arms are affected, an oversize pressure cuff may be used on the thigh or calf to measure the blood pressure. If you can't avoid the blood pressure to be taken on the arm, make sure that the cuff is inflated only 10mm/Hg above the systolic pressure (this is the point at which the pulse stops) and that only manual equipment is used – automated equipment inflates generally to a very high pressure, which is held for a prolonged period.

- To take care of minor injuries, always carry an alcohol swab, topical antibiotic, and a band-aid with you.

- Avoid piercing or tattoos on the arm, back, or chest.

Avoid Heat

- Avoid very hot showers.
- Avoid hot packs and/or ice packs on your arm, back, and chest.
- Avoid traditional massage on the arm, chest, and upper back area. Note: Manual lymph drainage is not considered to be a form of massage.
- Avoid sunburn; while in the sun, use sunscreen, cover the arm with appropriate clothing or a dry towel.

Exercises

- Discuss proper exercises and activities with your therapist.

- Avoid movements that over strain; should you experience discomfort in your arm, reduce the exercise activity and elevate your arm.

- Avoid heavy lifting.

Nutrition (see also 3.7.1)

- Maintain healthy body weight.
- Keep your diet well balanced; most nutritionists recommend a low-salt and low-fat diet, high in fiber.
- Eating too little protein in the hope to have a positive effect on lymphedema is not recommended and may cause health problems. Reducing the protein intake will not reduce the protein component in lymphedema.

Travel (see also 3.7.2)

- Avoid mosquito-infested regions.
- Wear an additional bandage on top of your compression sleeve when traveling by car, train, or air. Incorporate frequent stops, or get up from your seat frequently, and elevate your arm(s) as often as possible.

See your doctor if you

- Have any signs of an infection, such as fever, chills, or red and hot skin.
- Notice any itching, rash, fungal infections, or any other unusual changes on the skin.
- Experience pain, or an increase in swelling in your fingers, hand, arm or chest.

Lower Extremity

Certain activities may trigger the onset of lymphedema or may exacerbate the symptoms of existing lymphedema. Individuals affected by lymphedema and those at risk for developing it (everyone who has undergone lymph node excision and/or radiation treatments) should observe the following precautions, which are based on decades of experience and knowledge of clinical experts in the field of lymphedema management.

Skin Care

- Keep your skin meticulously clean and check frequently for any cracks, fungal infections, or rashes.
- Moisturize your skin daily, especially after taking a shower or bath. Use appropriate ointments or lotions.
- Dry your skin thoroughly with a soft towel after taking a shower or bath; do not scrub.
- If you undergo radiation therapy apply the ointments recommended by your physician to any radiation redness on your skin and avoid direct exposure to sunlight.
- Avoid cosmetics that irritate the skin.

Clothing, Jewelry, Compression Stockings

- Avoid clothing that is too tight, such as underwear, socks, or stockings that restrict.
- Do not wear tight jewelry and avoid elastic bands around your ankle.
- Wear your compression stocking or pantyhose all day, and if necessary, apply your bandages at night. Use rubber gloves when you put on your compression garment. See your certified lymphedema therapist (CLT) at least every six months to check the condition of the garment.

Avoid any Injuries to the Skin

- Shaving: use an electric razor to remove hair from the leg or abdominal area; do not use razor blades.
- Nail care: you should keep your toenails short but be careful cutting your toenails, do not cut the cuticles.
- Pets: be careful playing with your pets (scratches).
- Mosquito bites: wear insect repellents and avoid mosquito-infested areas.

- Injections on the swollen leg (or the leg at risk), in the buttocks on the affected side, or in the abdominal area should be avoided whenever possible.
- To take care of minor injuries, always carry an alcohol swab, local antibiotic, and a band-aid with you.
- Do not walk barefoot and wear solid shoes to avoid ankle injuries.
- Avoid piercing or tattoos on the leg or the abdominal area.

Avoid Heat

- Avoid very hot showers and hot packs and/or ice packs on your leg or the leg at risk.
- Avoid traditional massage on the leg and the lumbar area. Note: Manual lymph drainage is not considered to be a form of massage.
- Avoid sunburn; use sunscreen and cover the leg with appropriate clothing or a dry towel.

Exercises

- Discuss proper exercises and activities with your lymphedema therapist.
- Avoid movements that over strain, should you experience discomfort in your leg, reduce the exercise activity and elevate your leg.
- Elevate your leg as often as possible.

Nutrition (see also 3.7.1)

- Maintain healthy body weight and keep your diet well balanced. Most nutritionists recommend a low-salt and low-fat diet, high in fiber.
- Eating too little protein in the hope to have a positive effect on lymphedema is not recommended and may cause health problems. Reducing the protein intake will not reduce the protein component in lymphedema.

Travel (see also 3.7.2)

- Avoid mosquito-infested regions.
- Wear an additional bandage or stocking on top of your compression garment when traveling by car, train, or air. Incorporate frequent stops, or get up from your seat frequently, and elevate your leg(s) as often as possible.

See your doctor if you

- Have any signs of an infection, such as fever, chills, or red and hot skin.
- Notice any itching, rash, fungal infections, or any other unusual changes on the skin.
- Experience pain, or an increase in swelling in your toes, foot, leg or lower body quadrant.

Support Groups

Lymphedema support groups can be a helpful tool for individuals who share the common diagnosis of lymphedema to come together and share coping tips, experiences, news, and most importantly, emotional support.

The help and information received in lymphedema support groups may take the form of providing and evaluating relevant information on treatment modalities, self-care, relating personal and listening to other's experiences, and establishing social networks.

While providing important emotional support, support groups are more than just a safety net for the patient; in fact, they can even improve the physical health and wellness of participants. Members of an established support group not only serve as educators for individuals newly diagnosed with lymphedema, but also inform the public about this condition, engage in advocacy, or can serve as a clearing house for disseminating news on important advancements or therapies.

Most support groups are facilitated by individuals who have personal experience with lymphedema, and became advocates for others. These groups may have regularly scheduled meetings, or exchange information via online forums.

There are also professionally operated support groups, which are facilitated by professionals who do not share the problem of the members, such as lymphedema therapists, social workers, psychologists, or members of the clergy. In these settings, the facilitator controls discussions and provides other relevant information; such professionally operated groups are often found in hospitals or lymphedema treatment centers.

Lymphedema support groups can be found using an Internet search; a number of institutions provide lists of support groups, such as the National Lymphedema Network, the Lymphatic Network and Research Foundation, and others.

3.7.1 Nutritional Aspects

There is no special diet for lymphedema. An accepted nutritional approach in the management of lymphedema is to follow a balanced diet, which, in addition to physical activity and exercises, promotes weight loss. Excessive weight contributes to greater demands on the lymphatic systems ability to drain fluid from the tissues; weight control therefore positively affects lymphedema.

Studies indicate that obesity does have an influence on lymph fluid level and extremity volume[37, 38]. Obesity and overweight often worsen the symptoms associated with lymphedema; a balanced nutrition, and portion-appropriate diet contributes to reducing the risk factors associated with lymphedema.

A balanced and healthy diet including whole grains, fish, fruits, and vegetables, and avoiding fatty foods will greatly assist in achieving and maintaining a healthy weight without restricting the intake of important nutrients and vitamins. "Crash" diets or diets which restrict certain food groups and nutrients are not advisable.

Protein: There is a common misconception that lymphedema may be positively affected by limiting protein intake. Although lymphedema is defined as an accumulation of water and protein in the tissues, it is essential to understand that lymphedema cannot be reduced by the limitation of protein ingestion, which can even be potentially dangerous.

Fluids: Limiting fluid intake does not reduce the swelling; the established protocol among lymphedema professionals is not to restrict fluid intake. In fact, fluids are typically encouraged, good hydration with water is essential for basic cell function, and especially important before and after lymphedema treatment to assist the body in eliminating waste products.

Salt: Lymphedema, like other forms of edema, appear to benefit from a low salt diet, but clear scientific evidence is lacking[39]. The *2020-2025 Dietary Guidelines for Americans* recommend that Americans consume less than 2,300 milligrams (mg) of sodium per day as part of a healthy eating pattern. However, the amount of salt in the typical North American diet is estimated to be 3,400 mg per day.

Excess salt in the diet is linked with high blood pressure, which increases the risk of heart disease and stroke. In addition, osteoporosis, stomach cancer, kidney disease, kidney stones, and generalized edema are linked to chronic excess salt intake[40].

Vitamins and other supplements: There are no vitamins, food supplements, or herbs that have been proven to be effective in the reduction of lymphedema. In the US, dietary supplements are regulated as food, not drugs. Pre-market approval by the Food and Drug Administration (FDA) is not required unless specific disease prevention or treatment claims are made. Because there is no requirement to review dietary supplements for manufacturing consistency, and no specific standards for dosage or purity exist, there may be considerable variations within the products marketed as dietary supplements.

Individuals affected by lymphedema are often in need of additional vitamins and supplements, especially if they battle recurrent episodes of infections. To determine which supplements and vitamins are beneficial, patients should consult with their physicians and/or nutritional specialist.

3.7.2 Traveling with Lymphedema

Travel involves spending prolonged periods of time sedentary, and does present a risk of developing swelling, which is often observed by travelers having swollen feet and ankles during and after spending long hours sitting in a car, bus, train, or aircraft. This is frequently observed by individuals with an intact lymphatic system; extended times of inactivity coupled with a compromised lymphatic system, can have even more serious consequences.

Narrow seats, minimal legroom, a low cabin pressure (versus atmospheric pressure), dehydration, and other factors present a particular challenge for lymphedema patients, regardless if the upper or lower extremity is affected.

There are a number of research articles available on the topic of air travel and lymphedema, some demonstrating the onset of lymphedema during and after travel, others denying it[(41,42)]. Any lymphedema developing, or worsening because of travel-related issues is one too many; although traveling with lymphedema presents some risks, and requires a little more planning, it should not discourage lymphedema patients from taking a trip.

Being aware of particular travel-related risk factors enables patients to take precautionary measures before, during and after traveling, and help to avoid the onset of swelling, or the exacerbation of existing swelling in lymphedema.

One of the most important measures involve wearing of compression garments to counter the negative effects on lymphedema during air travel.

The National Lymphedema Network (NLN) states in its position statement on air travel that "Individuals with a confirmed diagnosis of lymphedema should wear some form of compression therapy while traveling by air. Individuals at risk for developing lymphedema should understand the risk factors associated with air travel and should make a decision to wear compression based on their individual risk factors."[(43)]

Wearing compression on the extremity affected by lymphedema, or an extremity being at-risk of developing it, effectively counters the effects of low aircraft cabin pressure and venous pooling in the extremities as a result of prolonged sitting, by increasing the pressure inside the tissues.

Other precautionary measures:

- Moisturize your skin prior to travel.
- Wear a well-fitting compression garment.
- Ask your therapist if it is advisable to apply an additional sort-stretch bandage on top of your garment.
- Avoid lifting and carrying heavy bags; use rolling suitcases and ask someone to place your luggage in the overhead compartment.
- Wear comfortable and loose clothing and shoes you have worn previously.
- Stay hydrated and drink plenty of water, cabin air is dry.
- Move around the cabin frequently.
- Use your legroom to perform decongestive ankle and toe exercises; if possible, request an exit seat for more legroom.
- Elevate your arm as often as possible.
- Leave your compression garment on until you reach your final destination.

3.7.3 How to Clean Compression Materials

Compression bandages and garments used in the management of lymphedema should be properly washed on a regular basis, so skin cells and oils won't become trapped in the fibers of the bandages and damage the integrity of the textile.

Compression Garments

Sleeves and stockings are generally worn from morning until night time, and although compression stockings are constructed of strong elastic and durable materials, they stretch out after about twelve hours of wearing, especially in areas of increased stretch, such as the knee or elbow, which may result in pooling of edema fluid in those areas. It is advisable to have more than one garment, which should be worn alternately to allow the elasticity to recover, and to prolong their effectiveness.

Daily washing of compression garments not only cleans them but also helps to restore and retain their elastic properties. Frequent washing does not harm compression garments if done properly; manufacturers generally include care instructions with their compression sleeves and stockings.

Garments may be machine or hand-washed; the water temperature can range between cool and warm, but should not be colder than 86 degrees Fahrenheit, or warmer than 104 degrees Fahrenheit. Darker-colored garments should be washed in cool water.

Mild soaps or detergents should be used, free of bleach, chlorine, fabric softeners, or other laundry additives. Some manufacturers offer special garment washing solutions, which are formulated to help extend the life of elastic garments.

Although compression garments may be machine dried (no heat), air-drying is the preferred method. It is important not to pull, squeeze or wring out the residual water from the garment; rolling up the compression garment in a towel and gently squeezing the towel before laying them out to dry, speeds up the drying process.

Whether garments are line-dried or laid flat to dry, exposure to direct sunlight should be avoided, and the garment should be turned inside out. It is recommended to place a towel on a drying rack and lay the garment on top to dry. If hanging the garment directly on a rack or pole to drip dry, the weight of the water could stretch the garments, causing them to fit improperly.

The elastic fibers of a compression garment will break down with wear, which makes it necessary to replace them periodically. While proper care will increase the lifespan of garments, they will need to be replaced about every six months, or when the garment shows signs of wear that could adversely affect the compressive properties of the garment. As a rule, if the garment no longer returns to its original shape after washing, has runs or holes in the material, or no longer feels compressive, it should be replaced.

Compression Bandages

Daily washing of short-stretch compression bandages is recommended. Tubular stockinette, padding bandages and gauze are not designed to be washed and should be replaced once they become soiled.

Short-stretch bandages may be machine or hand-washed; the water temperature should be warm (up to 140 degrees Fahrenheit); boil-wash (up to 200 degrees Fahrenheit) is possible for very dirty bandages. The unrolled bandages should be placed in a mesh laundry bag in order to protect the fabric during the washing cycle.

Compression bandages should not be ironed. For soaps, detergents and drying procedures, please refer to compression garments, the procedures are the same.

Short-stretch bandages can be washed up to 50 times without losing their elasticity. While proper care will increase the lifespan of short-stretch bandages, they will need to be replaced about every six months, or when the bandages loose their stiffness and recoil.

References

(1) Zasadzka E et al. Comparison of the effectiveness of complex decongestive therapy and compression bandaging as a method of treatment of lymphedema in the elderly. Clin Interv Aging.2018; 13: 929–934.Published online 2018 May 14.doi:10.2147/CIA.S159380

(2) Michopoulos E et al. Effectiveness and Safety of Complete Decongestive Therapy of Phase I: A Lymphedema Treatment Study in the Greek Population. Cureus.2020 Jul; 12(7): e9264.Published online 2020 Jul 19.doi:10.7759/cureus.9264

(3) Document, C., (2020) "The diagnosis and treatment of peripheral lymphedema: 2020 Consensus document of the International Society of Lymphology",*Lymphology*53(1), p.319.doi:https://doi.org/10.2458/lymph.4649

(4) Nudelman J. How to find a qualified lymphedema therapist.Lymphatic Education and Research Network. Accessed July 2022. (www..lymphaticnetwork.org/living-with-lymphedema/find-a-lymphedema-therapist)

(5) Lasinski B et al. A systematic review of the evidence for complete decongestive therapy in the treatment of lymphedema from 2004 to 2011.PM R2012 Aug;4(8):580-601.doi: 10.1016/j.pmrj.2012.05.003.

(6) Fu MR, Deng J, ArmeR J. Putting Evidence Into Practice: Cancer-Related Lymphedema: Evolving Evidence for Treatment and Management From 2009-2014.CJON2014, 18(6), 68-79.doi: 10.1188/14.CJON.S3.68-79

(7) Ganeswara LM et al.Effect of complete decongestive therapy and home program on health- related quality of life in post mastectomy lymphedema patients.BMC Womens Health.2016; 16: 23.Published online 2016 May 4.doi:10.1186/s12905-016-0303-9

(8) Kwan ML, Cohn JC, Armer JM, Stewart BR, Cormier JN. Exercise in patients with lymphedema: a systematic review of the contemporary literature. J Cancer Surviv 2011;5(4):320-336. PMID: **22002586**.DOI:10.1007/s11764-011-0203-9

(9) Schmitz KH, Ahmed RL, Troxel AB, et al. Weight lifting for women at risk for breast cancer-related lymphedema: a randomized trial. JAMA 2010;304(24):2699–2705. PMID: **21148134**.DOI:10.1001/jama.2010.1837

(10) Kiriko A, Tetsuya T, et al.Postural differences in the immediate effects of active exercise with compression therapy on lower limb lymphedema. Support Care Cancer.2021; 29(11): 6535–6543. Published online 2021 Apr 29.doi:10.1007/s00520-020-05976-y

(11) Schmitz KH, Troxel A, et al. Physical Activity and Lymphedema (The PAL Trial): Assessing the safety of progressive strength training in breast cancer survivors. Author manuscript; available in PMC 2010 May 1. Published in final edited form as: Contemp Clin Trials. 2009 May; 30(3): 233–245.Published online 2009 Jan 8.doi:10.1016/j.cct.2009.01.001

(12) Schreiver I, Hesse B, Seim C. et al. Distribution of nickel and chromium

containing particles from tattoo needle wear in humans and its possible impact on allergic reactions.*Part Fibre Toxicol*16,33 (2019). https://doi.org/ 10.1186/s12989-019-0317-1

(13) Ross J, Matawa M. Tattoo-Induced Skin "Burn" During Magnetic Resonance Imaging in a Professional Football Player. A Case Report. Sports Health.2011 Sep; 3(5): 431–434.doi:10.1177/1941738111411698

(14) Position Statement of the National Lymphedema Network on the Diagnosis and Treatment of Lymphedema (https://www.mylymph.com/2018/03/08/the-diagnosis-and-treatment-of-lymphedema-position-statement-of-the-national-lymphedema-network/).Accessed May 2022

(15) The International Lymphedema Framework's Best Practice for the Management of Lymphoedema (BP PAGESfinjune8 bQ5 (lympho.org). Accessed June 2022

(16) Lymphedema Therapists' Dosing of CDT in Breast Cancer Survivors with Lymphedema. Published December 2017 on the Internet Journal of Allied Health Sciences and Practice (IJAHSP). ("National Survey of Lymphedema Therapists' Dosing of Complete Decongest" by Katie M. Polo, Peter J. Rundquist et al. (nova.edu). Accessed June 2022

(17) National coverage determination for pneumatic compression devices (http://www.cms.gov/medicare-coverage-database/details/ncd-details

25&ncdver=1&NCAId=63&IsPopup=y&bc=AAAAAAAAAgAAAA%3D%3D&). Accessed July 2022

(18) Feldman JL, Stout NL, Wanchai A, Stewart BR, Cormier JN, Armer JM. Intermittent Pneumatic Compression Therapy: A Systematic Review. Lymphology 45(2012) 13-25

(19) Zaleska, M., Olszewski, W. L., & Durlik, M. (2014). The effectiveness of intermittent pneumatic compression in long-term therapy of lymphedema of lower limbs.*Lymphatic research and biology*,*12*(2), 103–109. https://doi.org/10.1089/lrb.2013.0033

(20) Cormier JN, Rourke L, Crosby M, Chang D, Armer J. The surgical treatment of lymphedema: a systematic review of the contemporary literature (2004-2010).Surg.Oncol. 2012 Feb;19(2):642-51.

(21) International Lymphedema Framework Position Document. Best Practice for the Management of Lymphoedema – 2ndSurgical Intervention. (https://www.lympho.org/wp-content/uploads/2021/09/Surgery-final.pdf). Accessed June 2022

(22) Cormier JN, Cromwell KD, Armer JM. Surgical Treatment of Lymphedema: A Review of the Literature and a Discussion of the Risks and Benefits of Surgical Treatment. 24 No. 2 – LymphLink Reprint

(23) Brorson H, Svensson H, Norrgren K, Thorsson O. Liposuction Reduces Arm Lymphedema Without Significantly Altering The Already Impaired Lymph Transport. Lymphology 31 (1998) 156-172.

(24) Granzow JW, Soderberg JM, Kaji AH, Dauphine C. An Effective System of Surgical Treatment of Lymphedema.Ann Surg Oncol. 2014 Apr;21(4):1189-94.

(25) Park, K. E., Allam, O., Chandler, L., Mozzafari, M. A., Ly, C., Lu, X., & Persing, J. A. (2020). Surgical management of lymphedema: a review of current literature. *Gland surgery*,*9*(2), 503–511. https://doi.org/10.21037/gs.2020.03.14

(26) Loprinzi CL, Kugler JW, Sloan JA, et al. Lack of effect of coumarin in women with lymphedema after treatment for breast cancer. N Engl J Med 1999; 340(5): 346-50

(27) UK Dermatology Clinical Trials Network's PATCH Trial Team, Thomas K, Crook A, et al. Prophylactic antibiotics for the prevention of cellulitis (erysipelas) of the leg: results of the UK Dermatology Clinical Trials Network's PATCH II trial. *Br J Dermatol.* 2012;166(1):169-178. doi:10.1111/j.1365-2133.2011.10586.x

(28) Stanford Medicine. Anti-inflammatory drug effective for treating lymphedema symptoms. (https://med.stanford.edu/news/all-news/2018/10/

anti-inflammatory-drug-effective-for-treating-lymphedema-symptoms.html). Accessed June 2022

(29) Bower JE, Woolery A, Sternlieb B, Garet D. Yoga for cancer patients and survivors. Cancer Control. 2005 Jul;12(3):165-71. Doi: 10.1177/107327480501200304. PMID: 16062164

(30) Moadel AB, Shah C, Wylie-Rosett J, Harris MS, Patel SR, Hall CB, Sparano JA. Randomized controlled trial of yoga among a multiethnic sample of breast cancer patients: effects on quality of life. J Clin Oncol. 2007 Oct 1;25(28):4387-95. doi: 10.1200/JCO.2006.06.6027. Epub 2007 Sep 4. PMID: 17785709.

(31) Narahari SR, Aggithaya MG, Thernoe L, Bose KS, Ryan TJ. Yoga protocol for treatment of breast cancer-related lymphedema.*Int J Yoga*. 2016;9(2):145-155. doi:10.4103/0973-6131.183713

(32) Ferguson CM, Swaroop MN, Horick N, Skolny MN, Miller CL, Jammallo LS, Brunelle C, O'Toole JA, Salama L, Specht MC, Taghian AG. Impact of Ipsilateral Blood Draws, Injections, Blood Pressure Measurements, and Air Travel on the Risk of Lymphedema for Patients Treated for Breast Cancer. J Clin Oncol. 2016 Mar 1;34(7):691-8. doi: 10.1200/JCO.2015.61.5948. Epub 2015 Dec 7. PMID: 26644530; PMCID: PMC4872021

(33) Nudelman J. Do No Harm: Lymphedema Risk Reduction Behaviors. J Clin Oncol. 2016 Sep 1;34(25):3109-10. doi: 10.1200/JCO.2016.67.9928. Epub 2016 Jun 13. PMID: 27298412

(34) Jeffs E, Purushotham A. The prevalence of lymphoedema in women who attended an information and exercise class to reduce the risk of breast cancer-related upper limb lymphoedema. Springerplus. 2016; 5:21. DOI: 10.1186/s40064-015-1629-8. PMID: 26759760; PMCID: PMC4703592

(35) Fu MR, Chen CM, Haber J, Guth AA, Axelrod D. The effect of providing information about lymphedema on the cognitive and symptom outcomes of breast cancer survivors. Annals of Surgical Oncology. 2010 Jul;17(7):1847-1853. DOI: 10.1245/s10434-010-0941-3. PMID: 20140528

(36) Lymphedema risk reduction practices.NLN Medical Advisory Committee-

Lymphnet. org, 2012

(37) Fu MR, Axelrod D, Guth AA, et al. Patterns of Obesity and Lymph Fluid Level during the First Year of Breast Cancer Treatment: A Prospective Study.*J Pers Med.* 2015;5(3):326-340. Published 2015 Sep 3. doi:10.3390/jpm5030326

(38) Helyer LK, Varnic M, Le LW, Leong W, McCready D. Obesity is a risk factor for developing postoperative lymphedema in breast cancer patients. Breast J. 2010 Jan-Feb;16(1):48-54.. doi: 10.1111/j.1524-4741.2009.00855.x. Epub 2009 Nov 2. PMID: 19889169.

(39) Dawson R, Piller NDiet and BCRL: facts and fallacies on the web. Journal of Lymphoedema, 2011, Vol 6, No 1

(40) Get the Scoop on Sodium and Salt. American Heart Association (www.heart.org/en/healthy-living/healthy-eating/eat-smart/sodium/sodium-and-salt). Accessed June 2022

(41) Casley-Smith JR, Casley-Smith JR. Lymphedema initiated by aircraft flights. Aviat Space Environ Med. 1996 Jan;67(1):52-6. PMID: 8929203

(42) Co M, Ng J, Kwong A. Air Travel and Postoperative Lymphedema-A Systematic Review. Clin Breast Cancer. 2018 Feb;18(1):e151-e155. doi: 10.1016/j.clbc.2017.10.011. Epub 2017 Oct 19. PMID: 29157874

(43) Position Statement of the National Lymphedema Network on airtravel (https://lymphnet.org/position-papers). Accessed June 2022

Index

A

B

C

D

E

F

G

H

Q

R

S

T

U

V

W

Y

Visit Lymphedema Blog (www.lymphedemablog.com) and

Lymphedema Guru on Facebook

Printed in Great Britain
by Amazon

25805714R10106